Insulin M

True life cases

Vincent Marks

Caroline Richmond

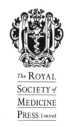

The ROYAL
SOCIETY of
MEDICINE
PRESS Limited

© 2007 Royal Society of Medicine Press Ltd

Published by the Royal Society of Medicine Press Ltd
1 Wimpole Street, London W1G 0AE, UK
Tel: +44 (0)20 7290 2921
Fax: +44 (0)20 7290 2929
Email: publishing@rsm.ac.uk
Website: www.rsmpress.co.uk

British Library Cataloguing in Publication Data

A catalogue record for this book is available from the British Library

ISBN 978-1-85315-760-0

Distribution in Europe and Rest of World:
Marston Book Services Ltd
PO Box 269
Abingdon
Oxon OX14 4YN, UK
Tel: +44 (0)1235 465500
Fax: +44 (0)1235 465555
Email: direct.order@marston.co.uk

Distribution in the USA and Canada:
Royal Society of Medicine Press Ltd
c/o BookMasters Inc
30 Amberwood Parkway
Ashland, OH 44805, USA
Tel: +1 800 247 6553/+1 800 266 5564
Fax: +1 419 281 6883
Email: order@bookmasters.com

Distribution in Australia and New Zealand:
Elsevier Australia
30-52 Smidmore Street
Marrikville NSW 2204, Australia
Tel: +61 2 9517 8999
Fax: +61 2 9517 2249
Email: service@elsevier.com.au

Typeset by Saxon Graphics Ltd

Printed in Great Britain by J H Haynes & Co Ltd, Sparkford

Contents

Foreword *Nick Ross*   v

Preface   vii

About the authors   ix

Acknowledgements   x

1. Kenneth Barlow, England: the first documented case   1

2. Herr Breslau, Germany: a brutal killing   7

3. William Archerd, USA: a serial matrimonialist killer   9

4. Claus von Bulow, USA: the first televised trial   19

5. Dolores Christina Miller, USA: why did she bother
   to kill a dying man?   51

6. Beverly Allitt, England: the nurse who killed babies   55

7. Jane Wagstaffe, England: was it suicide?   77

8. Maria Whiston, England: the "insulin between the toes" case   81

9. Susan Shickle, England: "It wasn't me, it was him"   95

10. Noburo Kato, Japan: a botched murder   101

11. Deborah Winzar, England: a case of wrongful conviction?   103

12. Vicki Jensen, USA: a heinous crime   133

13. Colin Bouwer, New Zealand: Professor of Psychiatry and
    murderer   135

14. Elaine Robinson, Wales: a bizarre death   157

Appendix   165

Further reading   177

Index   181

Foreword

Many people died to make this book possible.

Poisoning used to be all the rage. Back in the days when people routinely died young, and for unexplained reasons, it was relatively simple to spike somebody's food. Doctors didn't help. In the time of Plato and Pythagoras, disease was thought to result from supernatural forces. Even when it dawned on Hippocrates, Galen and the like that illness had physical causes, they put it down to imbalances of humors. This was not very funny for their patients. Right up into the 18th and 19th centuries, anyone who could afford a physician was likely to endure ridiculous misdiagnosis and painful, dangerous treatments not far removed from voodoo.

But all this credulous nonsense was great for poisoners. So long as medicine was stuck with superstition, who could say for sure whether your mother-in-law's black bile was out of balance with her phlegm or if you'd laced her drink with deadly nightshade? Antimony, copper, arsenic, lead, opium, cyanide and hemlock were all known to the Ancient Greeks – considering they thought ill-health was inflicted by the gods, they spent a lot of time finding ways to invoke it for themselves. Nero, in particular, was notorious for disposing of unwanted members of his family at the supper table.

By medieval times a host of toxic plants had been identified, and Chaucer was describing in his *Canterbury Tales* how a would-be murderer got from a "pothecary", *"Some poison that he might his rattes quell ..."* Quelling rats was always a good excuse for keeping some malevolent chemicals to hand. So much was known about poisons that *The Book of Venoms* of 1424 is almost a modern textbook on toxicology. In Italy the Borgias raised poisoning to a new art form, with professional poisoners offering themselves for hire – a practice that soon spread to Spain and France, prompting King Louis XIV in 1662 to ban the sale of many toxic substances and to set up a small detective force to investigate poisonings and root out the assassins. In England Queen Elizabeth I survived several poisoning plots and had her food checked by official tasters.

In fact, popular dread of poisoning probably greatly exceeded its real frequency, though, since nobody could tell the difference, many deaths from natural causes – like that of Napoleon Bonaparte – were ascribed to murder while, doubtless, many murders went undetected. Come the 19th century, fear of crime was stoked by the newly emergent newspapers, and chemists became obliged to have a Poisons Book to keep track of who bought what. Mostly it was husbands killing wives and wives killing husbands; poisons were easier to come by than divorce, and generally there was no point in poisoning someone unless you were married to them. As an added bonus, death was often slow and usually horribly painful.

But, bit by bit, science came to poop the poisoner's party. First came reliable tests for arsenic, and then, after Dr Crippen was sensationally caught fleeing to Canada and hanged for the murder of his wife in 1910, a Poisons Act swept most dangerous substances from the shelves, and, even more significantly, doctors were required to examine anyone who died unexpectedly.

Accordingly, the early 20th century saw a large number of prosecutions, and would-be killers had to be more cautious. Too many people got caught through old favourites such as arsenic and cyanide. If you wanted to get away with murder, it was wise to look for something new – something that might go undetected by a post-mortem. Ricin or thallium, perhaps, or better still, as this book shows – and it is as gripping as any crime thriller but splendidly educational too – *insulin.*

Nick Ross
TV and radio presenter; journalist and conference moderator

Preface

Insulin was probably the first of the miracle drugs discovered during the 20th century. It transformed type 1 diabetes – a more rapid, and certainly fatal, illness than cancer – almost overnight from a killer to a disease with which a patient could live a full and active life for 60 years or more. The down-side of insulin is that it can also kill you – either by accident or deliberately, whether by suicide or murder. It does so by reducing the amount of glucose in the blood to a level that is unable to sustain brain function. This happens very rarely when insulin is used properly, but not infrequently when it is deliberately misused.

The first recorded case of attempted suicide by insulin was in 1927, just 5 years after it had first been used to treat diabetes, and long before it became widely available to the public. By 1963 there were still only 13 cases of suicide by insulin known to medical science. All of the earliest cases survived – probably because the doses of insulin used were rather small compared with those used by later successful suicides and because, unlike most conventional poisons, insulin is not actually poisonous to the tissues. It usually causes death only when the blood glucose level stays low for 12 hours or more. This is rare, but does not prevent crime fiction writers choosing insulin as a murder weapon more often in books and plays than in real life – mainly because of the difficulty of detecting and proving it, as the cases described in this book demonstrate.

The first case of murder actually proved to be caused by insulin anywhere in the world occurred in England in 1957, and even then death was not due to the insulin itself but to the victim drowning whilst she was incapacitated by hypoglycaemia (low blood glucose). Since that time I have been able to collect, through personal knowledge or from scientific papers, records of about 50 other cases of murder or attempted murder by insulin, many of them in children and elderly people. Its use has been suspected in many more – sometimes with dire consequences for the accused.

I first became interested in insulin, and its effect in overdose, when I was working at the National Hospital for Nervous Diseases in London in

1957 and was called upon to diagnose and treat patients suffering from a rare disorder of the pancreas that causes them to go into coma from hypoglycaemia. That interest persists to the present day.

Although I had been involved with patients who had committed various offences whilst they themselves were suffering from hypoglycaemia, my introduction into the realm of murder by insulin began with a phone call from America. I was asked if I was prepared to help in the case of Claus von Bulow, who was on trial for the attempted murder of his wife, an extremely wealthy heiress. Since then I have been involved with many other cases in which insulin was, or was thought to have been, involved. I presented them some 6 years ago to a medicolegal audience in a scientific paper, but without any of the human background.

I realized that my writing style was not necessarily conducive to easy reading, and so recruited the help and advice of my co-author, Caroline Richmond, a distinguished medico-scientific journalist

Here we present – in many cases for the first time and in a form that we hope will be intelligible to a readership with an interest in crime and science – the best documented cases on record of murder, attempted or alleged murder, or manslaughter by insulin, many of which I was personally involved with. In the non-personal cases I have drawn largely or entirely on information available in the biomedical literature or the media at large, but only where there was sufficient information to make them interesting. This has meant omitting some cases that we know about but that are so poorly documented as to not be worth describing here.

The first case we describe is the Barlow case, which is widely accepted as the first in which murder by insulin came to trial. Subsequently, we have adopted a chronological approach as this enables us to illustrate how the methods of investigating hypoglycaemia and their use in providing crucial evidence have evolved, and avoids the need for repetition.

The facts relating to the cases described in the text are true, although in some cases the names of people have been changed to preserve their anonymity or because their full names are not recorded or available. The opinions expressed, except when quoted verbatim or specifically ascribed to others, are ours alone.

In order to help the reader with no previous knowledge of diabetes, blood glucose or insulin, we have included a glossary that describes them and the methods used in their measurement and detection. Reference to the glossary is not strictly necessary, but we hope that it may enhance the enjoyment of readers with an interest in the science as well as the criminality of the various cases.

Vincent Marks

About the authors

Vincent Marks

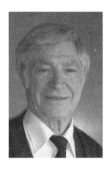

Vincent Marks went to Oxford on a scholarship to study medicine just after the Second World War. He became a world authority on hypoglycaemia early in his career, during which he was Professor of Clinical Biochemistry at the University of Surrey in Guildford, where he was also Dean of the Science Faculty and Founder of the Medical School. He is one of the pioneers of immunoassay and founder of the biotech company, ClifMar Associates, amongst others. He is a former President of the Association for Clinical Biochemistry and former Vice-President of The Royal College of Pathologists. He is one of the world's leading authorities on the measurement of insulin and has extensive specialist knowledge of medical research, including clinical chemistry and nutrition. Investigators worldwide call upon his expertise whenever a crime, or suspected crime, involves insulin or hypoglycaemia.

Caroline Richmond

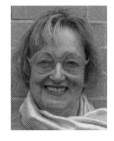

Caroline Richmond has had three careers: as a laboratory scientist in pharmacology and neurosciences; as a book editor; and as a science writer and medical journalist. She is a respected obituary writer for the *British Medical Journal*, *The Independent* and *The Guardian*, and also writes for *The Oldie* magazine. She founded HealthWatch, which campaigns for evidence-based medicine.

Acknowledgements

This book would not have been possible without the support I have received from various colleagues over the years in research into the causes, diagnosis and treatment of hypoglycaemia. Chief amongst them are Professor Frank Clifford Rose, whose encouragement led to the production of our joint monograph on the subject of hypoglycaemia in 1965; the late Professor Ellis Samols, who introduced me to immunoassay; and Dr Derrick Teale, who ran the immunoassay laboratory in Guildford that produced results used in many of the cases and with whom I collaborated in research into the nature and diagnosis of hypoglycaemia over a period of more than 30 years. I want especially to thank Lewis Marks QC, who read the text and made many useful and helpful suggestions. Finally, I would like to thank Nick Ross for writing a foreword.

Vincent Marks

1 Kenneth Barlow, England: the first documented case

On the morning of 4th May 1957, just after 2 am, Dr David Price, a forensic pathologist, was called by the GP to the home of Elizabeth and Kenneth Barlow in a residential suburb of Bradford, Yorkshire. The story was that Kenneth Barlow had discovered his wife unconscious in the bath at about 11.20 pm the previous night and called his own doctor, who diagnosed her as dead. Kenneth, a 38-year-old state registered nurse, was currently unemployed. He had married Elizabeth 11 months earlier and was, to all outward appearances, living happily with her and his 10-year-old son by his first wife.

According to Kenneth, Elizabeth had had tea at about 5 pm on the day of her death. Shortly afterwards she announced that she was tired, and went to bed. When Kenneth came to bed at about 9.30 pm he found that Elizabeth had vomited on the bed. Together they changed the sheets. She put on some pyjamas but took them off because she said she felt too warm and decided to take a bath. Kenneth lay on the bed and went to sleep at about 9.45 pm to the sound of the bath running. When he woke up at around 11.20 pm Elizabeth had not returned to bed. When he went into the bathroom he found her submerged beneath the water. He tried to lift her out but did not have the strength to do so. Nevertheless, he held her head above the water until all the water had run out of the tub. He said he then tried artificial respiration by *"pressing on her abdomen"* as he was unable to lift her from the bath. Only after this was unsuccessful did he run next door to his neighbours, who had a telephone, and ask them to call a doctor.

The family doctor arrived only 10 minutes later and found Elizabeth in the empty bath in a position simulating natural sleep. He did not touch her beyond ascertaining that she was dead. With such an unexpected death he felt it necessary to call the police, who in turn called Dr David Price, who was on-call as Home Office forensic pathologist. His main job was as consultant pathologist at the nearby Beckett Hospital in Barnsley.

Dr Price suspected from the beginning that this was not a natural death for two reasons. First, death from drowning in a domestic bath in a previously perfectly healthy 32-year-old woman is rare. Secondly, but even more telling, was the 110 ml (a small cupful) of water that remained in the cavity where the crook of Elizabeth's arm abutted the side of the bath. This made Kenneth's story that he had tried to resuscitate her difficult to accept and, consequently, his account of the events suspicious.

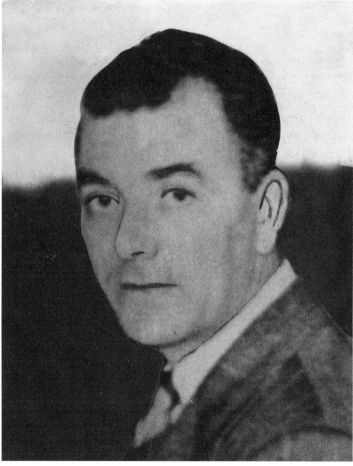

Figure 1 Kenneth Barlow. Photograph reproduced with permission from Topham Picturepoint.

Meanwhile the police had made a thorough search of the house and uncovered nothing very much except two vomit-stained pillow cases in the bathroom wash-hand basin, a set of sweat-drenched pyjamas in the bedroom and a couple of used syringes in the kitchen. Because of the latter, the police searched the house for vials (bottles) of insulin or other injectable medications but found none.

Dr Price began a post-mortem examination in the local mortuary at 5.45 am, only 3½ hours after he first saw Elizabeth's body and 6 hours after she had died. He noted that her pupils were widely dilated and that there was bloodstained froth in her nose, mouth and throat. Samples of her lungs, when examined under the microscope, were bulky, congested and wet. They also revealed fluid retention and small haemorrhages, confirming the initial diagnosis that death was caused by drowning. Apart from this, he found no abnormalities, but did observe that Elizabeth was 8 weeks pregnant. In addition, Dr Price took the precaution of collecting blood from a number of different sites in the body as well as some urine from the bladder to send to the poisons laboratory, just in case she had been poisoned. The samples were examined by Dr Alan Curry of the North-Eastern Forensic Science Laboratory, who went on to become one of the most distinguished directors of the UK's forensic science service nationwide.

Dr Curry found none of the common poisons or abortion-causing substances in any of the samples he examined. Nevertheless, Dr Price and his senior police colleagues remained convinced that Elizabeth had been rendered unconscious before she drowned, and they considered the possibility that she had been injected with insulin. This would explain her excessive sweating and dilated pupils before death.

Four days later, on 8th May, the decision was made to re-examine Elizabeth's body more thoroughly and under bright light. On this occasion, and with the benefit of a magnifying glass, two hypodermic injection sites were identified in each buttock. Dr Price removed these, with their surrounding tissues, and stored them in a refrigerator until he could find a scientist with the expertise and facilities to undertake an insulin test. The methods available at the time were comparatively crude by today's standards and could only be performed by a handful of specialist laboratories. They relied on finding the dose that caused hypoglycaemic convulsions in mice, and comparing the sample with standardized samples containing known amounts of insulin. It was the method used at that time to measure the strength of pharmaceutical insulin extracted from animal pancreases before releasing it for use by patients.

Dr MR Gurd of the research laboratories of the Boots drug company, which was one of three British manufacturers of insulin at the time, undertook to perform the test. Dr Gurd did not, however, hold out much hope of success. He thought the technique might not be sensitive enough to detect the small amount of insulin that would be found in the tissues of someone who had received an insulin injection.

Dr Gurd did, in fact, find easily measurable quantities of insulin in extracts of the tissues taken from Elizabeth's buttocks. For comparison, Dr Price had removed tissues from other corpses, which Dr Gurd treated in the same way. As he expected, he found no trace of insulin in them. So, the findings from Elizabeth were clearly abnormal and therefore highly suspicious.

On 5th July, two months after Elizabeth's death, Dr Gurd reported that he had been able to recover from three separate samples of Elizabeth's buttocks a total of about 84 units of insulin, enough to keep two insulin-dependent diabetic patients going for a whole day. Elizabeth did not have diabetes, nor had she been prescribed insulin.

On the basis of this evidence, Kenneth Barlow was confronted by the police on 26th July, whereupon he admitted injecting Elizabeth, but not with insulin. He said he had, with her permission and collaboration, injected her with ergometrine, a drug used legitimately in obstetrics at the conclusion of a delivery and by lay people, when they could get hold of it, to try to induce an abortion, and which was clearly illegal. He was unaware that this possibility had already been considered – and ruled out – by the toxicological examination conducted by Dr Curry on Elizabeth's body immediately after her death and, subsequently, by examination of the needles and syringes found in the kitchen.

Between the time that Kenneth Barlow was charged with murdering Elizabeth and his case coming to court, a new, much more sensitive and precise method for measuring insulin in body fluids had become available. This involved measuring the uptake of radioactive glucose by muscle tissue (a rat's diaphragm) incubated at body temperature for several hours in a flask containing a sample of the patient's blood serum diluted in a special type of saline. The rate of glucose uptake by the muscle is directly proportional to the amount of insulin present in the incubating fluid. The only exponent of this technique in Britain at the time was Dr Peter Wright of Guy's Hospital, London, with whom I was collaborating in the investigation of non-diabetic patients with hypoglycaemia and neurological symptoms.

Dr Curry asked Dr Wright to examine the extracts made from Elizabeth's buttocks. His results confirmed those of Dr Gurd. To ensure that the methods he was using measured insulin and not just something like it, Dr Wright used four different techniques to improve the specificity. One of these techniques used an antibody against insulin made in guinea pigs and called an anti-insulin antiserum. The effect of this was to neutralize any insulin present in the extract by binding to it and making it unavailable to the rat diaphragm. In Elizabeth Barlow's case it abolished the insulin effect produced by the untreated extracts. This use of insulin antibodies foreshadowed their use in the immunoassay first employed in the Archerd case (see page 15), and indeed in all subsequent cases of murder by insulin that have come to trial. No longer would it be possible to sustain the myth that insulin is the perfect weapon because it cannot be detected after death.

Among the other substances tested for by Dr Curry were phenolic preservatives used in commercial insulin preparations. None was found, but he explained this by their rapid disappearance from injection sites, unlike insulin, which remains there acting as a depot for up to 24 hours, depending on the type of insulin used. He also measured the glucose content of the blood Dr Price had removed from Elizabeth's heart, as it would surely be low if she had died of an overdose of insulin. Imagine his surprise therefore when, instead of finding a low blood glucose concentration, he found it abnormally high. To someone less expert than Dr Curry this might have been the end of the matter. He knew, however, that scientists had previously observed a rise in the concentration of glucose in blood that was collected from the right side of the heart of people who had died a violent death but that it was usually low in blood collected from leg veins or from the left side of the heart.

With the assistance of various forensic pathologists who collected blood from victims of violent deaths for him to analyse, Dr Curry confirmed the earlier discovery that blood glucose levels in blood from the right side of the heart do not reflect the blood glucose concentration in the rest of the body after death. As a result the investigating team were not put off pursuing an otherwise very strong case by what, on the face of it, seemed at first to be an insuperable obstacle.

With Dr Gurd's results to go on there seemed so little doubt that Elizabeth had been injected with insulin that the prosecution proceeded to trial even before Dr Wright's results became available. The prosecution recognized that some people deliberately inject themselves with insulin for a variety of reasons, including suicide, but as it is difficult for anyone to inject themselves in their buttocks, it was obvious to them that someone else had done it and that that person was Kenneth.

Before the trial it emerged that earlier in the year Kenneth had told a fellow employee at the hospital where he was working about an accident his wife had suffered the previous September. On that occasion, he claimed, he had found her collapsed in a hot bath and rescued her by removing her from it. He had also, it transpired, boasted to fellow workers over a period of 2 years how easy it would be to kill someone with insulin since it was undetectable in the body after death. There appeared to be no motive for killing his wife apart from the rather tenuous one that he did not want her to have a child.

Kenneth vehemently denied the charge of murder but at his trial at Leeds Assizes in December 1957 could not explain the insulin found in Elizabeth's body apart from suggesting that she had administered it herself. The absence of insulin vials and of any insulin in the two syringes that had been found, together with the improbability of self-administration into the sites where the insulin was found, all militated against this possibility.

The jury found Kenneth Barlow guilty, on the evidence, and Mr Justice Diplock sentenced him to life imprisonment on 13th December 1957. He was released from prison 26 years later, in 1984, still maintaining his innocence.

Although usually described as the first case of murder by insulin to lead to conviction, Elizabeth Barlow did not in fact die from an insulin overdose, although it played a crucial role in her death. The amount injected into her was sufficient to render her unconscious and whether she would or would not have died had Kenneth left her long enough will never be known. It is probable that he had expected her to die quicker than she did and so he made the decision to drown her – which he did. Had he left her in her bed, she might well have been dead in the morning or at least have suffered irreversible brain damage and all of the insulin he had injected would have been absorbed into her bloodstream and destroyed. There would have been no 'smoking gun' for the pathologists and toxicologists to find and there would have been no case against him.

2 Herr Breslau*, Germany: a brutal killing

Frau Breslau*, a 32-year-old housewife, was already dead when Dr Levethal* arrived at her bedside on the evening of 4th January 1959. She had lived for several years in an apparently stable marriage in a small house in Bonn in Germany with her husband Wilhelm*. Dr Levethal, a local practitioner with no particular forensic experience, had been called to see her by Wilhelm, who told him that his wife suffered from an overactive thyroid and suggested that this had caused her heart to fail. This can undoubtedly happen – although it is rare, as it was even in the 1950s, when diagnosis was much less accurate and treatment for thyrotoxicosis (as the condition is called) was much less readily available than it is today. Nevertheless, the doctor accepted this explanation and, without examining the body, certified death from heart failure due to thyrotoxicosis.

Frau Breslau was buried 3 days later, on 7th January, without an autopsy. There the matter would have ended had not a close relative raised the possibility that she had not died from natural causes. Frau Breslau's body was exhumed 2 days later. A post-mortem examination by a skilled and knowledgeable forensic pathologist revealed a body with numerous bruises, gashes to the scalp, and injection sites on the thighs and arms. The pathologist, who was probably aware of the Barlow case, which had already been written up just a few months earlier in the *British Medical Journal* of 12th August 1958, removed some of the tissues surrounding the injection sites. He sent them to the laboratory of Professor Ernst Pfeiffer at Frankfurt University for analysis for insulin. Professor Pfeiffer, one of Germany's leading specialists in diabetes, and later to become President of the University of Ulm, used a technique similar to that used by Dr Gurd (see page 3) rather than the more sophisticated one used by Dr Peter Wright in the Barlow case (see page 3). Nevertheless he found substantial amounts of insulin in the tissue extracts taken from several of the numerous injection sites – even though

---

*   Not his/her real name.

the body was already several days old. Confronted with the evidence, Wilhelm and his mistress gave full and complete confessions.

Wilhelm Breslau and his mistress had tried various methods of killing his wife during the 4 days preceding her death. She had, it appears, been persuaded to become drunk to the point of senselessness on New Year's Eve 1958, and as a result she vomited in the bathroom but survived. Less than 2 days later, between 4 and 5 am on the morning of 2nd January, the lovers hit her on the head with a beer bottle with sufficient force to knock her out. She recovered from this assault, and later that afternoon they injected her intravenously with, among other things, 5–10 ml (or about 1–2 teaspoonfuls) of a mixture of petrol and air. Even this did not kill her: neither did the barbiturates they gave her. Finally, on the evening of 3rd January, again at midday, and for a third time at 2 pm on 4th January, they injected her with insulin. They gave some intravenously and some by injection into the muscles of her thighs and arms. In all they admitted to giving her at least 400 units of insulin – enough to keep 10 typical insulin-dependent diabetic patients going for a day. Wilhelm's mistress was a registered nurse working in a hospital for patients with terminal illnesses and had stolen the insulin from there.

Although hypoglycaemia was probably the cause of Frau Breslau's death, the other injuries inflicted upon her undoubtedly contributed. At their trial Wilhelm and his mistress were both found guilty of murder and sentenced to life imprisonment.

This case illustrated, as had already been established in the Barlow case, that killing someone with insulin is far from easy. It is neither rapid nor, disconcertingly from the killer's point of view, undetectable after death.

3 William Archerd, USA: a serial matrimonialist killer

William Dale Archerd, also known as James Lynn Arden and by other pseudonyms, was found guilty on 15th March 1968 of murdering his nephew and two of his seven wives. These were probably not the only killings he committed. He was then 55 years old and had a varied past as salesman, erstwhile mental hospital attendant and serial matrimonialist. His wives had a habit of dying, and William had chosen insulin as the weapon to kill two, and possibly three, of them as well as his other victims. He presumably stole it, as for much of the time he was unemployed, but he could also have bought it over the counter as insulin was not a prescription-only drug and was freely available. Although his murderous career really began in 1947, it was only 20 years later, when he was arraigned for murder, that his earlier crimes came to light.

William had, it seemed, always wanted to be a doctor but, not having the opportunity, and possibly the ability, to pursue this career, spent some time during the early 1940s working as an orderly in a state mental hospital – and the next 25 years in a life of crime.

In 1950 some of his earlier misdemeanours caught up with him and he was sentenced to 5 years' probation after pleading guilty to illegal possession of morphine. The probation was revoked after he committed a second drug offence. He was sent to a minimum-security prison, from which he escaped a year later, in 1951.

After recapture he was sent to the high-security, and highly notorious, San Quentin jail, from which he was released on parole in 1953. San Quentin had been established in 1852 at Point Quentin, an island off Marin County in San Francisco bay, as an answer to the rampant lawlessness in California at that time. California's only gas chamber and death row for all condemned male inmates were located at San Quentin and it was possibly there that William was launched into serious crime.

The story begins when William contacted the police on 24th July 1956 to report an alleged robbery at his home in Los Angeles. He said that two robbers had come to his home, armed with guns and hypodermic syringes, which they had used to inject both him and his current (third) wife, Zella,

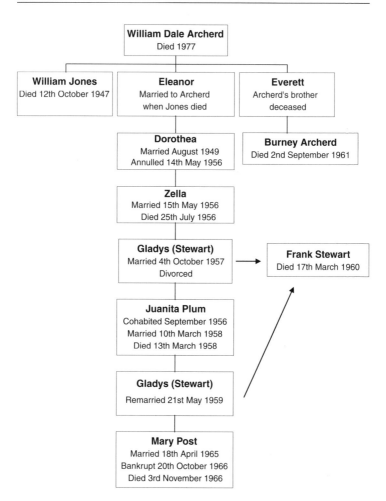

Figure 2 Chronology of Archerd's victims.

in the buttocks. They made off with $500 but none of Zella's jewellery, which was on full view in her bedroom. At the scene of the crime the police initially found two puncture wounds in Zella's buttocks – later amended to four after examination of photographs taken of her after death. There were none in William's.

Zella was dizzy but not comatose when the police arrived, and she corroborated her husband's statement about the robbers, although she never saw them, as they put a pillowcase over her head. After the police left she gradually lapsed into coma and had convulsions from which she died next day without regaining consciousness. During a search of the house and surroundings the police found a hypodermic needle in a bathroom drawer and a half-used vial of long-acting insulin in a nearby field.

The investigating police officer in Los Angeles, whose name was Sergeant Harry André, drew the coroner's attention to the insulin vial. However, because no poisonous substances were found in Zella's body and no method of measuring insulin was readily available except in research laboratories, he had no evidence that she had died from insulin poisoning. Zella's death was officially attributed to bronchopneumonia but suspicion remained, at least in Sergeant André's mind, that she might have been murdered.

The second death to come to the attention of the authorities was that of Juanita, William's fifth wife. She and William lived in Las Vegas, Nevada, where William had gone to live soon after Zella's death. Juanita was discovered in a coma on 12th March 1958 – only 2 days after she and William had married, and less than 2 years after Zella's death in Los Angeles. Like Zella, Juanita was taken to hospital but died only a few hours after being found and without regaining consciousness. Her doctors attributed her coma to a self-administered barbiturate overdose. This was not confirmed by blood analysis, as the methods for measuring barbiturates were too difficult to do routinely. She also had a low blood sugar for which there was no obvious medical explanation. In the light of what subsequently emerged, Juanita's coma was almost certainly due to insulin but, once again, the crucial test was not done.

William Archerd's name cropped up yet again, just over a year later when, having married for the sixth time, his new wife's ex-husband, Frank Stewart, died in a Nevada hospital on 17th March 1960. He had been taken there after having allegedly slipped on a banana skin in a toilet in the airport while he was on a business trip with William, and had struck his head as he fell. Frank never regained consciousness. William's account of Frank's accident was accepted. Despite the authorities' suspicion of dirty work, no criminal cause could be found to account for Frank's death.

Because both Juanita's and Frank's deaths had occurred in another state and consequently outside Sergeant André's jurisdiction, there was little he could do about them. Nevertheless he reported his suspicions about William to the Nevada police authorities but, despite the strong circumstantial evidence pointing to wrongdoing, they were unable to find sufficient evidence to implicate William in Stewart's death. Once again, as no one had measured Frank's blood glucose level while he was unconscious, the authorities never considered the possibility of insulin overdose.

William Archerd's name next came to Sergeant André's attention a year and a half later when he read a newspaper account of Burney Kirk Archerd, William's nephew, who died following a hit-and-run traffic accident in Nevada. William had taken his nephew to hospital on 21st August 1961 in a semi-comatose state. Burney was complaining of a sore hip and scalp and, on examination, the pupil of one eye was dilated. This is common after a head injury, but, with the benefit of hindsight, it could have been caused by William putting atropine into one of Burney's eyes to produce inequality in pupil size to feign a head injury. Burney became fully comatose during the evening and night of 23rd August, shortly after a visit from Uncle William. He never regained consciousness and died 10 days later, on 2nd September 1961.

The only laboratory abnormality recorded in Burney's clinical notes was a low glucose concentration in his cerebrospinal fluid (CSF). This had been collected as part of the investigation of his coma believed to be due to a head injury. No particular significance was attached to the low CSF glucose concentration and – by implication – low blood glucose concentration until after Burney's death. The pathologist who conducted Burney's autopsy was aware of the Kenneth Barlow case (see page 1), and later said that he had considered the possibility that his coma was due to insulin. But he had no means of proving it, since any insulin, even if it had been there originally, would long since have gone. Burney's death was put down to the car accident that had brought him into hospital.

Sergeant André then drew William's record to the attention of Sergeant White of the Los Angeles homicide squad. Sergeant White had been charged with investigating fatal road accidents in a large area surrounding the city, and his involvement in this case played a crucial role in unravelling the story. He became further involved after he had investigated, and disproved, a fraudulent claim by William for damages following a road accident he said he had been involved in, but which had been deliberately staged by him in collusion with others, including his then current girl friend, Stella Morrin, who was fortunate enough not to marry him. There was, however, still no definite evidence linking William with the deaths of Frank, Burney, Zella or Juanita – though suspicion ran high.

William then changed his name to James Lynn Arden. Things came to a climax when his seventh wife, a romantic novelist called Mary Brinker Arden, died on 2nd November 1966, allegedly as a result of head injuries sustained in a road traffic accident, 18 months after her wedding. Lieutenant White, as he now had become, was assigned the job of investigating Mary's death, which was far from straightforward.

William and Mary had lived together for about a year after their marriage but parted when she became bankrupt. William then returned to live with his sixth wife, Gladys. After her car accident on 28th October, Mary got in touch with William, who, after she had returned home from the hospital, went to her house to console her. Two days later Mary was admitted to hospital in a coma and she died the next day without recovering consciousness. Blood tests showed she had a very low blood glucose level and that some barbiturates were present.

Here was yet another suspected murder by insulin but with no hard evidence to go on. For reasons that are far from clear, neither Lieutenant White nor any of his forensic medical advisers appears to have known that, 6 years earlier, in 1960, an exquisitely sensitive method had been developed for measuring insulin in blood and other body samples.

The technique, called radioimmunoassay, was to earn one of its inventors, Rosalyn Yalow, the 1977 Nobel Prize for Physiology or Medicine. Unfortunately, her co-inventor, Sol Berson, who died in 1972 aged 54, could not participate in the award, as it is never given posthumously.

Radioimmunoassay rapidly became accepted as the best, and at that time was the only sensitive and reliable method for measuring insulin in blood and tissues at the infinitesimally low concentrations in which it occurs in the body even after criminal or suicidal use. Indeed, in 1963, 3 years before Mary's death described above, Ellis Samols and I had published our experience of immunoassay for investigating the cause of hypoglycaemia in patients with insulin-secreting tumours. Others, including of course Rosalyn Yalow and Sol Berson, were using it routinely to measure insulin in the blood of patients for research and other purposes.

Lieutenant White established contact with Dr Edward Arquilla, who was the Professor of Pathology at the University of California Los Angeles Medical Center, and was nearby. By coincidence, Dr Arquilla had himself, some years earlier, invented a technique for measuring insulin in blood and tissues using antibodies. It was not as sensitive or reliable as the radioimmunoassay method devised by Berson and Yalow and consequently was less widely used.

Immunoassay uses antibodies to measure substances in blood in a test tube. It can also be used to detect substances in thin sections of tissue removed at operation or autopsy without measuring their actual concentration. This technique is known as immunohistology and identifies substances that react with the antibody to the exclusion of everything else – or so the theory goes. In those early days, before its complexity was fully appreciated, immunohistology was relatively crude. It could create artefacts and was not as reliable as many people supposed – especially in the forensic situation. Even so, it provided

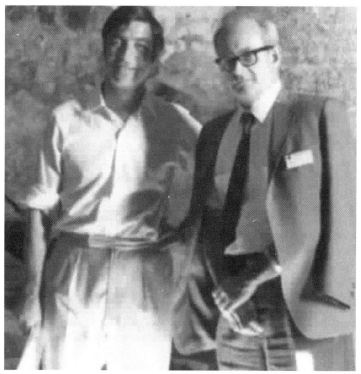

Figure 3 Vincent Marks with Sol Berson, co-inventor with Rosalyn Yalow of radioimmunoassay. Taken at Château de Chillon during a conference in Geneva, 1969.

useful information for research and sometimes for diagnostic purposes in the clinic.

At the police department's request, Dr Arquilla applied an immunohistological technique using his own insulin antiserum to thin slices of Burney's brain that had been collected at post-mortem and preserved. They reacted with the insulin antibodies whereas normal brain tissues did not. Dr Arquilla was also given some of Mary's brain from which he made extracts that he injected into mice. He showed that they lowered blood glucose concentrations in the mice more than did similar extracts made from normal brain. From this he concluded that the samples contained abnormally high quantities of insulin. Dr Arquilla's results did not become available, however, until after William had already been charged, on 27th July 1967, in Los Angeles, with the murders of Zella, Burney and Mary. Indeed, Dr Arquilla did not even receive the samples for analysis until the day the trial itself had begun. This was on 4th December 1967, by which time the police had interviewed 400 people in extensive investigations. Among them was Dorothea, William's second wife, from whom he was divorced just 1 day before he married Zella. Until the investigations proved otherwise, Zella was believed to be William's first victim.

Although Archerd was not specifically charged with the offences, the court allowed evidence to be heard "to show common plan or scheme" that William had used insulin to murder Juanita, his fifth wife, the ex-husband (Frank Stewart) of his sixth wife and a friend (William Jones). This decision was made after Dorothea, who was a nurse and still alive, had told the police about the death of William Jones. Jones had been involved in a moneymaking scam with William Archerd – who killed him by an insulin injection in 1947. Jones had, apparently, agreed to let William Archerd inject him with insulin as a cover-up for some of their illegal activities – which involved faking unconsciousness due to a head injury purportedly caused by a motoring accident – not knowing or appreciating the consequences of what he was doing.

Dr Grace Thomas testified at William's trial. She had been the psychiatrist in charge of Camarillo State Hospital at a time when William worked there and when insulin coma therapy for schizophrenia was in vogue. She told the court that the hospital records of all of his victims found alive were consistent with hypoglycaemia. Dr Robert Tranquada, Professor of Medicine and a well-known endocrinologist from the University of Southern California in Los Angeles, and who had written extensively on the investigation of hypoglycaemia, agreed with her.

William had waived his right to trial by jury and was found guilty by the presiding judge on three counts of first-degree murder for the deaths of Zella, Burney and Mary. On 6th March 1968, he was sentenced to death in the gas chamber of San Quentin State Prison. Later, in 1970, the California State Supreme Court confirmed the conviction. They also held that evidence that he had killed Juanita, Frank – the former husband of his wife at the time – and a friend (William Jones) was admissible as showing *"a common plan or scheme"*. A further 2 years later, in 1972, William's sentence was commuted to life imprisonment after the US Supreme Court had ruled that the death penalty was a *"cruel and unusual punishment"*. The US death penalty was subsequently re-instated in the USA in 1974 and the first post-Supreme Court execution took place 2 years later, although William himself escaped it.

With the benefit of hindsight, and subsequent knowledge of how insulin behaves in the body, it is unlikely that the results of the tests for insulin in the brains of Burney and Mary would stand up in court today since they were almost certainly artefacts. We now know that insulin cannot be accurately detected in the brain, as it is easily confused with related chemicals. Without these measurements that were used in court, there must be some uncertainty that what was undoubtedly a justified conviction would have been obtained. What is truly surprising is that even as late as 1966, when Mary died, none of the doctors looking after her – or for that matter those consulted by the police – knew about Yalow and Berson, radioimmunoassay or the dozens of papers that had been published describing its use for measuring insulin in blood.

William appears to have been motivated by greed throughout his career of crime. This was not established in every case but in some it seems pretty certain. Zella had been comparatively well off when he married her and he stood to gain from her death. Junita left an estate worth $40,000 but, unbeknownst to William, she had, shortly before she died, altered her will so that he got none of it. Frank Stewart had taken out $80,000 worth of accident insurance payable to William's aged mother and his former wife, Gladys, as beneficiaries in the event of his death whilst on his business trip with William. The insurance company, however, refused to pay out on the policy, not having been convinced that his death was accidental, so once again William left the scene empty-handed. William's nephew Burney had been awarded $8000 in compensation for the death of his father, and William had been named as trustee. After Burney's death none of the money could be found or accounted for. Mary was a successful author in her own right and, as her next of kin, William stood to inherit her estate, whatever it was worth, despite her bankruptcy.

William died of pneumonia in 1977 at the age of 65. The judge described him at the end of his trial as *"the most evil man of our times"*. This may have been something of an overstatement, but we know what he meant.

4 Claus von Bulow, USA: the first televised trial

In 1982, and again in 1985, Claus von Bulow was tried in a US court for the attempted murder of his wife by injecting her with insulin. He was found guilty at the first trial and sentenced to 30 years in jail. The conviction was quashed on appeal, and at a second trial he was, quite rightly, found innocent and acquitted since it was scientifically established that no crime had been committed.

Sunny von Bulow, or Martha as she was baptized, was the daughter of George W Crawford, who died when she was only 4 years old, leaving her a huge fortune. She had, early in life, come into the limelight by marrying two Europeans of very distinguished ancestry. Her first husband, an Austrian Prince, fathered her first two children. Her second husband, Claus von Bulow, had graduated from Cambridge at the early age of 19, practised as a barrister in Lord Hailsham's chambers, and then joined the late billionaire, J Paul Getty, who described him in his autobiography as *"my right arm"*. Claus had also been a member of the Danish Olympic Winter Sports Team in 1948 and had lived for many years, prior to his marriage, in his large home in London's Belgrave Square. After the marriage the couple ultimately settled in Sunny's two homes on New York's Fifth Avenue and in that renowned fortress of American "old money", Newport, Rhode Island.

Insulin can be used to commit suicide or even murder, as we have already seen, by inducing prolonged and eventually irreversible coma. It was, however, Claus's trial, the first to be televised live on American television, that brought insulin to the public's attention as a potential murder weapon.

There are four major episodes in Sunny's medical history during the last year of her life as a free-living individual that are germane to the story. She suffered two episodes of hypoglycaemic coma, and never recovered from the second but continued – and continues – to live in a persistent vegetative state. In addition, she was investigated in hospital in the middle of 1980 to try to determine why she had gone into hypoglycaemic coma just after Christmas 1979, and she had been admitted to Lennox Hill Hospital New York suffering from aspirin poisoning in early December 1980, 3 weeks before her final hypoglycaemic coma.

Claus's first trial was a travesty – the defence called virtually no expert medical evidence to rebut the false hypothesis that Sunny's hypoglycaemic comas were due to insulin. The prosecution called Dr George Cahill, undisputedly one of the world's authorities on hypoglycaemia, who was adamant at Claus's first trial that Sunny's comas were insulin-induced, though at the second trial, when confronted by conflicting opinions by authorities as eminent as himself, he was understandably less sure. The defence doctor at the first trial was Dr Milton Hamolsky. The defence virtually conceded that Sunny's comas were induced by an insulin injection – which they were not – and concentrated on raising doubt as to who gave it to her, posing the question: did she do it herself with suicidal intent or did Claus inject her with it? On the basis of some pretty damning circumstantial evidence, much of it no better than tittle-tattle relating to financial and emotional motivation, he was found guilty and sentenced to 30 years in jail.

It must be pointed out, as it was by the prosecution throughout the trial, that some of Sunny's medical history was supplied by Claus and was therefore potentially suspect as he was the prisoner in the dock. Some aspects of it were disputed by Sunny's two oldest children, Claus's stepchildren, who sided with their grandmother in accusing their stepfather of the attempted murder of their mother. Cosima, Claus's only daughter and Sunny's youngest, supported her father throughout his trials but, being in her early teens, was considered too young to give evidence.

It is no wonder that this scandal became a media circus with a concomitant decline in accuracy and fairness. Here we will concentrate on Sunny's medical history and the expert witnesses' evidence, which eventually established that as there had been no crime, there could not be a criminal.

Sunny's first admission to hospital for hypoglycaemia

Over the Christmas holidays of 1979, Sunny had apparently been unwell for a day or so before she was admitted to the emergency room of the Newport Hospital, Rhode Island. The history given by Claus to the doctor admitting her to the emergency room, and agreed by her, was that on 26th December, the evening prior to admission, Sunny – who had not been sleeping well – went to bed having drunk a substantial amount of alcohol. She slept through the night but did not feel well next morning

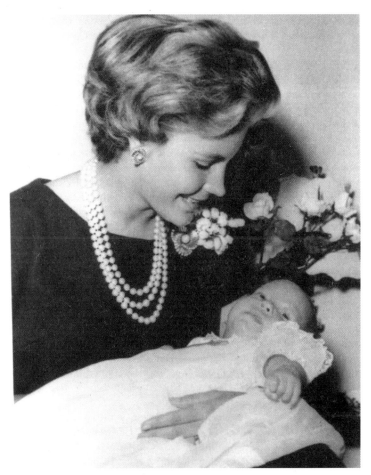

Figure 4 Sunny with Cosima in happier times.

and stayed in bed for most of the day, drinking only an occasional Coca Cola. By the afternoon of 27th December Sunny's breathing had become laboured, and at around 2 pm Claus called Dr Janis Gailitis, who was her family doctor and also a specialist in internal medicine at the nearby Newport Hospital. He only got the answering service. Dr Gailitis returned the call at about 3–4 pm, when Claus explained that his wife had been under intense emotional strain because of her eldest daughter's imminent departure for Austria and was not very well. Claus was not unduly worried about Sunny but he agreed with Dr Gailitis that he would keep a close eye on her. Some 3 hours later, at around 6 pm, Dr Gailitis received a frantic call from Claus saying that Sunny's condition had deteriorated rapidly and that her breathing was now very laboured.

Dr Gailitis arrived 15 minutes later, and entered Sunny's bedroom. He found her blue from lack of oxygen and struggling for breath. He attempted to find his stethoscope to listen to her chest but before he could do so Sunny started vomiting and stopped breathing. Dr Gailitis immediately swept the vomit out of Sunny's mouth with his fingers and felt for her pulse in her neck. Its absence indicated that Sunny's heart had stopped beating. Losing no time, Dr Gailitis began giving her external cardiac massage and mouth-to-mouth respiration, told Claus to call an ambulance and got someone to help him put Sunny on the floor, to make it easier to continue resuscitation. He saved her life by doing this.

By the time the ambulance arrived, Sunny's pulse had returned, albeit rather feebly, and she was breathing spontaneously. She was given oxygen in the ambulance and by 7.35 pm, when she arrived at the hospital, she was only slightly blue, but still deeply unconscious. In hospital Dr Gailitis continued the oxygen started by the ambulance crew. He set up a drip, giving her a steroid, Decadron (dexamethasone), to treat shock and an antibiotic, Mefoxin (cefoxitin). Her nose and face were still covered by vomit, and a blood test showed that she had accumulated acid in her body due to lack of oxygen. Consequently her comatose condition was attributed to lack of oxygen due to inhalation of vomit, and this was the view expressed by Dr Gailitis in court some 5 years later. It was almost certainly correct.

The blood test showed her blood glucose level was 2.3 mmol/L, considerably lower than normal (ordinarily it is within the range 3.5–10 mmol/L) but not low enough to cause coma. Dr Gailitis gave Sunny a bolus injection (ie a very rapid intravenous injection) of 25 g of glucose, as well as a glucose infusion at a modest 5 g/hour. Normally, a patient in hypoglycaemic coma of such short duration recovers consciousness within 10 minutes of such an injection, and often even before the needle is removed from the vein, but Sunny did not.

The first samples of blood and urine that were collected were tested for the presence of alcohol, barbiturates and drugs, and showed only aspirin. This was present at a very low concentration (0.33 mg/100 ml) in her blood and was only moderately high (245 mg/100 ml) in her urine. This is perfectly consistent with ordinary everyday use.

Shortly after admission to the emergency room, a surgeon, Dr Charles Hopper, was asked to look at Sunny's airways through a flexible fibre-optic bronchoscope. Dr Hopper did not find any foreign material or vomit in her trachea or bronchi but noted that there *"was a moderate amount of apparent acute tracheobronchitis and some secretion, which was aspirated* [sucked out]*"*. This means that her airways were inflamed, possibly from contact with vomit, and possibly from bronchitis.

The fact that Sunny was feverish and appeared to have a severe chest infection led her doctors, quite rightly in my opinion, to diagnose her as suffering from a severe toxic reaction, and to treat it accordingly. The diagnosis was subsequently supported by a blood test result from a sample taken when she was admitted. This showed a very high white blood cell count (of $18,400 \times 10^9$ per litre compared with a usual level of around $5000–10,000 \times 10^9$) 90% of which were of the polymorph variety – that is to say the variety that attacks bacteria. They are characteristically found in people with acute bacterial infections and are produced by the body as part of the natural immune response to those infections.

As is often the case when hospital clinical notes are examined later, long after the events, inconsistencies, including the timing of events and difficulties in reading the records – especially the signatures of the writers, if given at all – all came to light. The phraseology used in handwritten clinical notes, though adequate at the time for clinical purposes, does not necessarily meet the strict requirements of a court of law for forensic purposes, and too much reliance may later be placed on the typed clinical summary when the patient is discharged. In cross-examination Dr Gailitis was later to admit that the hospital notes were not up to much, though they were adequate for the purpose, which was to facilitate treatment. But for forensic use they were not as useful as they might have been.

No repeat blood glucose measurement was made in the immediate aftermath of the first glucose injection and Sunny continued to receive glucose by constant intravenous infusion at the slow rate of 5 g/hour. This amount is insufficient to meet the body's minimum needs for glucose in anyone whose liver is not supplying enough of it, but does serve to prevent the intravenous drip from becoming blocked by a blood clot.

Sunny's blood glucose concentration was not measured again until 11 pm. By then it had fallen to 1.1 mmol/L, which is abnormally low. Her level of consciousness was probably only slightly higher than it had been on admission. At midnight, when the glucose test result arrived back from the lab, she was, quite rightly, given a further bolus of 25 g of glucose intravenously and the glucose infusion rate through the venous drip was increased to 10 g/hour. By 3 am the next morning Sunny's blood glucose level had risen to 2.5 mmol/L, which is still below normal, and she was given a further bolus of 25 g of glucose and the infusion rate was increased to 20 g/hour.

The level and duration of Sunny's coma during this first episode was difficult to assess from the hospital notes. She is often portrayed in the media as having been in deep coma for many hours both before and after treatment with glucose began. This is incorrect. Dr Gailitis consulted an anaesthetist, Dr Tien, *"because* [he wrote in Sunny's clinical notes] *of her unconsciousness"*. A handwritten entry dated 27th December but untimed made by, or for, Dr Tien states, *"a 48 year old lady was intubated* [meaning that a tube was inserted into her throat in order to enable her to breathe]. *She was responsive to conversation,* [showed] *spontaneous respiration and* [her] *tidal* [breathing] *volume* [was] *330 cc* [millilitres]. *Assisted respiration is indicated"*. In other words, her breathing was dangerously shallow and she needed assistance from a ventilator.

Clearly Sunny could not have been unconscious in the strict meaning of the term if she was *"responsive to conversation* [the spoken word]*"*. This was, as far as can be made out, written before Sunny had been given glucose but could possibly have been written shortly after. Later, another handwritten clinical note records that, at 11.30 pm, Sunny was *"sleeping; easily aroused with stimulation"* and by 2–3 am on the morning of 28th December, 7 hours after admission, she was noted to be *"almost trying to sit up in bed, writing on pad, dozes off easily"*. These observations contradict the evidence given from memory by Dr Gailitis at the second trial, when he said that Sunny only regained consciousness 20–22 hours after admission to hospital. He was not actually there on the day after her admission, though he had done his duty the previous evening and saved her life by his prompt action at her bedside, and by prescribing steroids and antibiotics the moment she got in the door of the hospital.

By 4.30 pm on 28th December, while she was still receiving Decadron, antibiotics and glucose, Sunny had become completely lucid and was sitting up in a chair. From then on, her recovery was smooth – but slow, and therefore quite unlike that normally seen after an insulin-induced hypoglycaemic coma, where recovery is spectacularly fast unless brain swelling has occurred (and this only occurs after several hours of deep coma). Sunny's temperature and white blood cell count remained raised for a further 3 days – as it does in any severe infection. Hypoglycaemia can occur as a complication of such an illness but is relatively uncommon except in the elderly and people with certain metabolic abnormalities.

One week after her admission Dr Gailitis discharged Sunny from hospital with a diagnosis of aspiration bronchopneumonia after a cardio-respiratory arrest due to aspiration of vomit, and hypoglycaemia of undetermined origin. He strongly advised her to *"abstain from alcohol, barbiturates and tranquillizers in any form or fashion"*. He also stressed that it was important that the cause of her hypoglycaemia be investigated

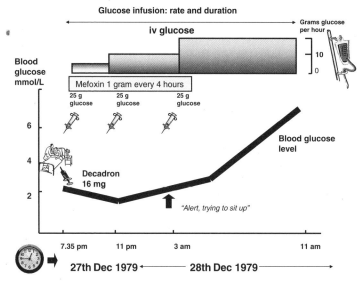

Figure 5 Time course of events during Sunny's first admission with hypoglycaemia 1979.

since the possibility of an insulin-secreting tumour had not been eliminated. He did not, unfortunately, consider the possibility that the hypoglycaemia was caused by infection or alcohol, although a consultant endocrinologist who saw her on 31st December, while she was still in hospital, wrote in the notes that she had "*probably hypoglycaemia related to alcohol and possibly barbiturates despite non-detectable ethanol* [alcohol] *level*". Unfortunately this suggestion was never followed up with the intensity it should have been. Though alcohol was probably not the primary cause of her hypoglycaemia on this occasion, it may have played some part and was almost certainly the cause of her second coma and admission to hospital a year later.

Sunny had a number of laboratory tests while she was in hospital during Christmas and New Year 1979, though probably fewer than would have been desirable. Perhaps this was because it was a holiday season. None of the tests carried out cast any real light on what had befallen her or caused her hypoglycaemia, which was quite clearly secondary to some other condition. No attempt was made to identify the bacteria that had caused her fever, high white cell count and pneumonia, which was put down to inhalation of vomit even though the evidence on this point was incomplete. Sunny was, after all, already blue from lack of oxygen when

Dr Gailitis arrived on the scene and before she had vomited. *"Vomiting"*, as Dr Daniel Foster, one of the experts called by the defence said in court, many years later, *"is as rare as hens' teeth"* in insulin-induced hypoglycaemia and he had never seen it in 30 years of specialist practice. It is, however, relatively common in people with hypoglycaemia from other causes.

Insulin was first measured in a sample of blood collected at midnight, after Sunny had already been shown to be hypoglycaemic and had been given ample amounts of glucose. As well as the glucose infusion, she had received the two 25 g boluses already mentioned, and a third one around midnight. Dr Gailitis said at trial that he could not be certain whether the sample sent for insulin assay was collected before or immediately after the third injection of glucose. In order to be clinically and forensically useful, it needed to have been collected before and whilst her blood glucose level was still low. This is why it is essential to measure the blood glucose concentration in any sample of blood submitted for insulin assay – a high glucose level would have shown that the sample was collected after the glucose injection, a low level would have put it before that injection.

Dr Milton Hamolsky, the local endocrinologist who testified at the first but not the second trial, stated that the sample was collected after the glucose injection. This was probably an educated guess, as there was no documentary evidence to support the statement, made because the result was normal (518 pmol of insulin/L; the usual range is 30–700 pmol/L). There is, unfortunately, no evidence that the glucose and insulin were measured on the same sample and, even more unfortunately, neither was C-peptide (see Appendix) – as would undoubtedly have be done in the best regulated circles.

Dr Hamolsky's assumption was probably correct and the first insulin assay result had been obtained on a blood sample collected after rather than before the glucose injection, making it of little use for diagnosis. Getting the sequence of blood collection for insulin assay and the injection of glucose in the wrong order is a relatively common mistake and one I have encountered on several occasions when investigating the cause of a patient's hypoglycaemia. So too is the failure to measure glucose in the sample of blood submitted for insulin assay, although without it the result is usually almost worthless both clinically and forensically.

A second plasma insulin measurement was made on blood collected from Sunny at about 7 am on 28th December, several hours after her blood glucose levels had been restored to normal and while she was still receiving intravenous glucose. The result, 388 pmol/L, was unremarkable.

Once again, regrettably, blood glucose and insulin levels were not measured from the same sample.

Amongst the causes considered for Sunny's hypoglycaemia were an insulin-secreting tumour (called an insulinoma) of the pancreas and sulphonylurea ingestion. Sulphonylureas are drugs that patients with maturity-onset (type 2) diabetes take to stimulate their own pancreas to secrete insulin. When taken by non-diabetics, or in overdose, they can produce hypoglycaemia and have been used to commit suicide and even murder (see the Bouwer case, page 135). Screening tests for sulphonylurea drugs were carried out on Sunny's blood collected 12 hours after admission but were negative. This was not altogether surprising, since not only were they unlikely, on purely clinical grounds, to have been the cause of her hypoglycaemia but the test used was far too insensitive to have detected them if they had been taken in anything but massive overdose.

Dr Gailitis took the precaution of asking Dr Marc Fellner, the local endocrinologist, to see Sunny and to advise on her condition. He considered it possible that she might have an insulin-producing tumour but, as already mentioned, thought it *"most likely* [that her] *hypoglycaemia was due to alcohol and barbiturates despite undetectable alcohol level"*. He further advised that the *"patient should have a 5-hour glucose tolerance test in future when she is well"*.

Sunny was discharged on 2nd January 1980 fully lucid and with "no neurological problems as a result of her illness, with strong advice *"to abstain from alcohol, barbiturates and tranquillizers in any form or fashion"*. In conversation with Dr Richard Stock, who had been Sunny's family doctor in New York City since 1965 and was a specialist in heart medicine, Dr Gailitis stressed the importance of getting follow-up studies done when she was back in New York to try to find the cause of Sunny's hypoglycaemic episode.

Sunny spent her holidays in Rhode Island but lived mainly in New York, and it was there that she was investigated in the spring and summer of 1980 to attempt to establish the cause of the hypoglycaemic episode she experienced over the Christmas holidays.

Interim investigations

Dr Stock arranged to admit Sunny to The Presbyterian Hospital in New York City on 21st April 1980 under his care in order to investigate the cause of her hypoglycaemia. She had been well since her discharge from Newport Hospital in January. Indeed, during the 30 years she had been his patient she had visited Dr Stock in his office only 16 times, and had received just nine house calls. Apart from the recent illness she had been in hospital only twice: once in 1967 for acute peritonitis, and once in December 1977 when she was 46, for a fractured hip. This is an unusual injury in someone as young as Sunny and is often associated with alcohol misuse, which she denied at the time. She was, as far as Dr Stock was concerned, in excellent health but did require investigation to determine the cause of the hypoglycaemia.

Sunny's notes made on admission to The Presbyterian Hospital record that *"in addition* [to the history obtained from the patient and from the referral letter], *the patient's mother, husband, and two children have noticed intermittent ataxia* [unsteadiness of gait], *slurred speech and drowsiness for 4–6 months"*. In other words, something had been going on since, or even before, the onset of her illness the previous Christmas. The admission notes go on to record that when *"examined by me* [Dr Stock] *at home last week the Rhomberg* [a test for balance] *was positive, she was unable to walk in a straight line and heel to knee and finger and to nose tests were ataxic* [hesitant and imprecise]. *She denies the use of drugs and takes alcohol in small amounts only"*.

The symptoms described by the family, and the clinical observations made by Dr Stock, are common in many diseases of the nervous system. They can, as everyone knows, also be caused by alcohol. Less well known is the fact that intermittent hypoglycaemia caused by an insulinoma can do the same. Since Sunny denied alcohol abuse and there was no evidence of serious neurological disease, Dr Stock, not unnaturally, opined for hypoglycaemia due to an insulinoma, and decided to enlist the help of Dr Kermit Pines, the hospital's endocrinologist.

A standard 5-hour glucose tolerance test was done before breakfast on the day after her admission to hospital for investigation. Sunny drank 100 g of glucose dissolved in water. Blood was collected from a vein at intervals for the next 5 hours and tested for its glucose and insulin content. The overnight fasting level of blood glucose was perfectly normal, and rose normally, but not excessively, after drinking the glucose solution. By 3 hours the venous blood glucose level had fallen to the very low level of 1.3 mmol/L and remained low for the next hour or so before gradually returning towards normal at 5 hours. Comments made at the time were *"glucose tolerance test is compatible with fasting or organic hypoglycaemia. Of interest is patient's lack of symptoms other than profuse perspiration and weakness at 3 and 4 hours"*.

A 72-hour fast was, at that time, generally considered to be the definitive test for ruling out the presence of an insulin-secreting tumour. Instead of doing this, the doctors withheld food from her for less than 48 hours. This failed to produce a fall in her blood glucose level to less than

3 mmol/L and did not produce an untoward effect on her. This was normal.

They then proceeded to do an intravenous tolbutamide test without feeding her. This test, which is no longer used as it is considered too unreliable, depends on the fact that tolbutamide stimulates the patient's own pancreas to secrete insulin. It is always done after an overnight fast, and in healthy people produces a temporary fall in blood glucose level that returns to normal within 2 hours of the injection. In patients with an insulinoma the fall in blood glucose is usually more prolonged and fails to return to normal by the end of the test. Sunny's blood glucose concentration fell to very low levels during the test and remained so.

There was no satisfactory explanation, except for the generally chaotic nature of the clinical notes, why the 10–60-minute blood glucose levels were not recorded during the tolbutamide test: they surely must have been measured. Fortunately they are not crucial to interpretation of the test result even in someone on whom the test had been done properly. The result obtained on Sunny, had the test been done properly with only an overnight fast, would have strongly suggested that she had an insulinoma, but because of the long period of fasting before the test was done, the result was uninterpretable. Surprisingly, despite the very low blood glucose levels observed, which were as bad as they were during the coma that took her into hospital over Christmas, Sunny experienced no serious side effects from the tolbutamide injection and certainly never lost consciousness.

Sunny had other tests, including an ultrasound scan, a computed tomography (CT) scan and an arteriogram of her pancreas. All were normal. The doctors rightly concluded that Sunny did not have an insulinoma but that still further tests should be done after she had spent some time at home. She was re-admitted for further investigation on 29th June in order to have glucagon and L-leucine tests, but in the event only the first was done and its result was normal.

The junior doctor who interviewed her and wrote the admission notes on this occasion observed that Sunny was *"a good historian"*. She (the doctor who carried out the interview writes neatly and legibly, so is very likely to have been a woman) also noted that on the *"night of admission* [Sunny] *had consumed large amount of alcohol"* and that there was *"Seconal* [secobarbital] *and tranquillizer use"*. This is virtually the only time in any of her hospital notes that information relating to alcohol and drug use appears to have come from Sunny herself rather than from her husband. This set of notes also record that *"since her previous admission* [8 weeks earlier] *she has been asymptomatic on a regime of low sugar and no alcohol"*.

An incidental laboratory finding, on this admission and on both the previous admissions, was that Sunny's red blood cells were larger than they ought to have been. This condition, called macrocytosis, is a feature of many illnesses, of which the most serious are vitamin B_{12} and folic acid deficiencies. However, appropriate laboratory tests had ruled out these possibilities. The most common cause is chronic alcohol abuse but this appears not to have been considered any further in view of Sunny's denial of drinking more than very occasionally.

Sunny was discharged from The Presbyterian Hospital in New York on 30th June with a final diagnosis of *"reactive hypoglycaemia"*. This was based exclusively on her response to the oral glucose tolerance test and the fact that an insulinoma had been ruled out. It is, however, an unsatisfactory diagnosis, but one that was extremely fashionable at that time, especially in the USA, where dubiously diagnosed "hypoglycaemia" had reached epidemic proportions. Indeed, Dr George Cahill, the chief expert for the prosecution in both of Claus von Bulow's trials, had in 1974 written a seminal article in the prestigious *New England Journal of Medicine* condemning "reactive hypoglycaemia" as a fashionable, but false, diagnosis. Neither he nor any of the other witnesses in the trial was to know that in 1986, just a year after the second trial had finished, an international panel of experts meeting in Rome would emphasize the uselessness and inappropriateness of the oral glucose tolerance test for diagnosing reactive hypoglycaemia. The panel effectively consigned the 5-hour glucose tolerance test to the rubbish bin as a clinical test for anything except diabetes.

The definition of reactive hypoglycaemia is a physiological over-reaction to a drink or meal containing glucose. Even when it does occur it is rarely severe enough to cause loss of consciousness or coma. Sunny had, however, been semi-comatose in December 1979, and if this had indeed been due to hypoglycaemia, it virtually ruled out the diagnosis of *reactive* hypoglycaemia she was given 6 months later in New York.

Sunny's second emergency admission

Sunny remained comparatively well for the rest of the summer and autumn of 1980 until she was admitted as an emergency to Lennox Hill, a local New York Hospital, under Dr Stock's care, at 12.15 am on 2nd December 1980.

She had been found confused and semi-conscious at home. On the assumption that she was again suffering from hypoglycaemia, a blood sample was sent to the laboratory to be tested for glucose and she was given a bolus injection of 25 g of glucose. This had no effect, and indeed

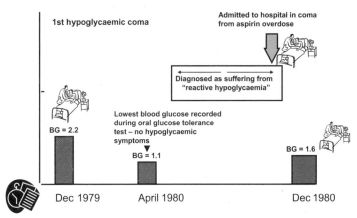

Figure 6 Chronology of events in Sunny's medical history 1979/1980. BG, blood glucose (in mmol/L).

her blood glucose before the injection was found to be normal (5.7 mmol/L). Hypoglycaemia was thereby ruled out as the cause of this particular coma. Instead it was attributed to an accident in which she had knocked her head and possibly suffered a bleed into her brain. A test carried out to determine whether her blood could clot properly showed that it did not. This, along with a head bruise, led to a provisional diagnosis of a haemorrhage into her brain caused by a head injury.

A neurosurgeon was asked to see her about her head injury and to treat her as he thought fit. She was transferred to The Presbyterian Hospital, where she had been investigated in the spring and which had facilities for dealing with a brain haemorrhage. She was admitted there with a provisional diagnosis of *"organic brain syndrome: metabolic acidosis, head trauma and coagulopathy"*. This was changed soon after she arrived to *"salicylate intoxication"* when the laboratory results from the Lennox Hill Hospital arrived showing that Sunny's blood had a very high aspirin concentration. This was above the level that would be fatal in over 50% of cases. She had clearly taken an overdose and was immediately treated for aspirin poisoning. She was infused with large amounts of fluid intravenously to wash the aspirin out of her body via urine. This was attended by a gradual fall in blood aspirin concentration and recovery of consciousness. She was discharged 4 days later fully recovered (at least physically) back to the care of Dr Stocks, her family practitioner, but without psychiatric support.

While she was in hospital Sunny was again observed to have larger red blood cells than normal. She was also noted to have iron-deficiency anaemia, which she had not had on previous occasions. This is normally associated with small rather than large red blood cells and was attributed, probably correctly, to bleeding into her intestine as a result of constant aspirin use. This suggestion was supported by tests carried out on her faeces, which confirmed the blood loss from her gut.

There is little evidence that any attempt was made to find out why Sunny had taken what several experts at Claus von Bulow's second trial estimated was at least 60 aspirin tablets in what can only be construed as a serious suicide attempt. In particular, no arrangements were made for Sunny to see a psychiatrist, even though she was obviously going through an emotionally traumatic patch. It subsequently emerged during both trials that on the morning of Sunny's admission to hospital for aspirin poisoning, Claus's mistress, an actress called Alexandra Isles, had delivered a package containing compromising material relating to their relationship to the von Bulows' New York apartment. This would undoubtedly have come to Sunny's attention. Dr Stock had recorded on 4th December, halfway through Sunny's 4-day stay in hospital, that Claus might be wanting a divorce, but he did not record the source of this information.

Third and final emergency admission to hospital

It is unclear exactly what happened to Sunny during the 16 days leading up to her next admission to hospital on 21st December 1980. She and Claus had moved from their New York apartment to their Newport home for the family Christmas holiday. On the morning of 21st December, after Claus had returned from walking the dogs at about 10 am, and Sunny had failed to materialize for breakfast, he and his stepson found her lying on her bathroom floor.

Immediately on making the discovery Claus called an ambulance, whose crew described finding Sunny lying on the bathroom's marble floor with a laceration to her upper lip, which had not been there the evening before, when Claus had last seen her close up. He had left their bedroom some hours earlier, as he always did, taking care not to disturb her as she lay asleep in her bed.

She arrived at the emergency room of Newport Hospital at 11.45 am deeply unconscious and with pinpoint pupils. At one stage she had no recordable blood pressure and her heart appeared to have stopped. Her body temperature was very low despite the warmth of the bathroom in which she had been found. It was established in court that her hypothermia was not due to the coldness of the room – the bathroom windows were, contrary to the impression many people gained from the gossip columns, shut – but was probably secondary to her hypoglycaemia, as is often the case.

Events immediately preceding the onset of her final illness suggest that she had gone to bed on the previous evening apparently quite well but having drunk alcohol. It subsequently emerged during the second trial that she had also taken amobarbital (Amytal), a powerful barbiturate sleeping pill, and at least eight propranolol tablets. These are used to bring down high blood pressure but also to prevent migraine attacks and had been prescribed for this purpose by Dr Stock the previous day.

Dr Gailitis, who had looked after her on her admission the previous Christmas, was away and Dr Gerhard Meier, who was deputizing for him, saw her. Dr Meier, though an experienced clinician, did not have a special interest in metabolism but was, familiar with Sunny through her medical notes. While taking a history from Claus, Dr Meier was interrupted by a nurse who told him that Sunny had stopped breathing. Dr Meier applied resuscitation and asked Dr Kenneth Laches, the Director of the Emergency Room, to collect a larger quantity of blood than usual from Sunny's thigh artery for various tests, including blood gases, glucose, insulin, alcohol and various drugs. Following resuscitation, Sunny's blood pressure, which had dropped to zero, gradually rose to normal. However, she continued to need artificial respiration for some time.

She was given 100 mg of Solu-Cortef (hydrocortisone) intravenously almost immediately on her admission to the hospital, followed by similarly large doses at 8-hourly intervals. This very powerful steroid is used for the treatment of shock of all sorts and helps to reduce swelling of the brain, a known complication of prolonged hypoglycaemic coma.

Apart from being unconscious, Sunny's other most obvious physical abnormality on admission to the emergency room was her coldness. Her body temperature was only 27.6 °C; ordinarily it is 35.5–37 °C. She was neither shivering nor blue from lack of oxygen, as she had been on her admission to hospital a year earlier. She was also noted to have a swollen right forearm, wrist and hand, but with no deformity, and Dr Austin White was asked for advice and treatment of this the following day. His opinion, given at the time, was that the swelling probably resulted from her lying in a single position for an extended period of time before being discovered.

Blood and urine were collected from Sunny shortly after noon, about half an hour after her admission, and sent to the laboratory for analysis. The report came back from the lab saying that the blood was markedly acidic (pH 7.24 compared with a normal pH of 7.4), had a low glucose concentration of 1.6 mmol/L (compared with a normal range of 3.5–6 mmol/L) and a low plasma potassium concentration of 2.2 mmol/L (compared with a normal range of 3.6–4.8 mmol/L). It also contained a trace of alcohol (9 mg/100 ml or 2.2 mmol/L). These results, apart from the blood glucose, received scant attention from the clinicians looking after her or those giving evidence at the first von Bulow trial. At the second they were to play a crucial role.

It was now after 12.00 noon and Sunny had so far received no treatment apart from Solu-Cortef and resuscitation. Immediately the blood glucose result became available, or possibly before, she was given 25 g of glucose by rapid intravenous infusion. With this she began shivering vigorously. It is an interesting, though not very well known, fact that people suffering from hypoglycaemia who are cold do not shiver, but start doing so the moment their blood glucose level is restored to normal. Though no particular attention was given to this observation at the time, it indicates very nicely that on this occasion hypoglycaemia was central to her illness. On the previous occasion, it was not, and was an incidental effect when her coma was due to lack of oxygen.

Sunny was given a further 25 g of glucose intravenously approximately 80 minutes after the first (at 1.50 pm) and an infusion of 10% glucose was commenced at the rate of 10 g/hour. At 1.10 pm instructions were given for insulin to be measured on the original blood specimen and also for various sulphonylurea drugs to be measured, but this instruction was apparently never carried out – to the considerable embarrassment of Dr George Cahill, who was asked about it during the trial and was unable to give a satisfactory answer.

No further blood glucose measurement was made until 7.00 pm, when it was abnormally high (14.5 mmol/L), though probably not dangerously so. By midnight Sunny had still not recovered consciousness although her blood glucose concentration had been normal or above for several hours. At 12.30 pm the following day, because of her continuing unconsciousness, she was referred to a neurosurgeon, Dr Jeremy Worthington. He recommended that Sunny be given Decadron to try to relieve intracranial tension – the build up of pressure due to fluid accumulation within the skull. This occurs in various conditions including head injury and prolonged hypoglycaemic coma. Sunny was given 6 mg – a large dose – of Decadron intravenously. It had no effect on her state of consciousness. An hour later, at 12.35 pm, she was given intravenous mannitol, whose function, like that of Decadron, is to reduce intracranial pressure. Because of her continuing coma, Sunny was then transferred from Newport Hospital to the Peter Bent Brigham Hospital, part of the Harvard Medical School in Boston, with a tentative diagnosis of irreparable brain damage caused by hypoglycaemia of unknown aetiology.

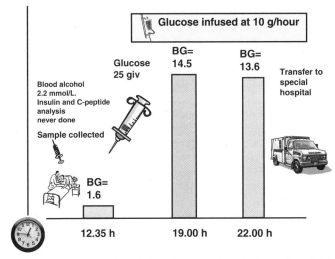

Figure 7 Events on the day of Sunny's second admission to hospital in a coma in December 1980. BG, blood glucose (in mmol/L).

Laboratory findings and how they led to a false suspicion of crime

It is worth noting that the first blood specimen collected from Sunny on her admission to the Newport Hospital was more acidic than it should have been (pH of 7.24 compared with a normal figure of 7.4) and contained far too little potassium (2.2 mmol/L compared with a normal range of 3.6–4.8 mmol/L). Her blood also contained alcohol. Its concentration of 9 mg/100 ml of blood (2.2 mmol/L), though low for most forensic purposes, was of very great medical importance and played a central role at the second von Bulow trial. The low plasma potassium concentration, which could have been explained by insulin-induced hypoglycaemia, it subsequently emerged was almost certainly due to Sunny's regular use of purgatives (sometimes, and foolishly, used as an aid to weight loss), a well-known and even more common cause of low potassium levels than insulin-induced hypoglycaemia.

Dr Meier instructed that some of the blood collected from Sunny when she was first admitted to the Newport Hospital should be sent to the laboratory to have its glucose and insulin content measured. The glucose measurement was made immediately but the sample for insulin and C-peptide (see appendix) content, and for the detection of antibodies against insulin, had to be dispatched to a commercial laboratory for analysis.

These tests were not performed in many hospital laboratories in 1980 but samples were sent either to specialist laboratories in university departments or to large commercial clinical laboratories.

Although Dr Meier issued his instruction at around 1.10 pm, about an hour after Sunny was admitted, the exact time at which the samples submitted for assay were actually collected is uncertain (this is an example of the difficulty of interpreting the notes). It seems likely, in fact, that the sample of plasma actually submitted for insulin and C-peptide assay was collected at 12.20 pm, about an hour before Dr Meier's instruction and presumably – though not certainly – before Sunny had been given the first injection of 25 g of glucose. The laboratory undertaking the assays did not measure the glucose content of the sample it received, so it is impossible to be certain that this was the same sample as the one that the local laboratory had found contained a low blood glucose concentration (another example of the difficulty of interpreting the notes).

Insulin and C-peptide tests, in 1980, took a few days to be reported and so treatment had to proceed without them. The laboratory report forms on which the results were relayed to the doctors stated only that the samples were collected on 22nd December and received in the laboratory on 23rd December, but this is unlikely to be correct. The samples were probably taken on the day of Sunny's admission, 21st December, rather than the day after.

The test to detect whether Sunny's blood contained antibodies against insulin showed it did not. Insulin antibodies are sometimes found in the blood of people who have been injecting themselves with insulin whether or not it was prescribed for the treatment of diabetes. Their presence in the blood of someone with a history of unexplained hypoglycaemia was, at that time, considered good evidence of surreptitious self-administration of insulin for one reason or another. We now know that this is incorrect.

The results of the insulin and C-peptide assays arrived after Sunny had already been transferred from the Brigham in Boston to The Presbyterian Hospital in New York, where she was receiving treatment for irreversible hypoglycaemic coma of undetermined origin and from which she neither recovered nor died but persisted in a vegetative state, as she remains even now (February 2007). They revealed that her plasma insulin level was high (1548 pmol/L) and her C-peptide level was normal (379 pmol/L). If they had both been high, this would have suggested a tumour that secreted insulin. However, the C-peptide level was low compared with that of insulin, leading the doctors to suspect that Sunny's hypoglycaemia was the result of an injection of insulin (exogenous insulin) rather than from any other cause.

The story of how this led to Claus von Bulow being charged with attempting to murder his wife with insulin is described in detail by Alan Dershowitz in his book *Reversal of Fortune* (1990) and will not be repeated here. Only at the second trial did it emerge that the high plasma insulin result, upon which the scientific case against Claus revolved, was almost certainly false.

Reversal of Fortune was subsequently made into a film that sensationalized the whole affair without examining closely the reason why there should never have been a trial at all since no crime had been committed. Sunny's illness that led to her irreversible brain damage was caused by her lifestyle, and in particular by her use of alcohol, painkillers, sleeping pills and purgatives – although her third admission to hospital was probably not a result of a deliberate suicide attempt, as the lawyers at Claus's first trial tried unsuccessfully to convince the jury it was. Her aspirin overdose, 3 weeks earlier, on the other hand, undoubtedly was a serious suicide attempt.

Expert evidence at the trials of Claus von Bulow

Following his conviction at the first trial, Claus changed his legal team and instructed Alan Dershowitz to pursue his appeal against conviction. After Mr Dershowitz had secured a ruling in April 1984 that the guilty verdict was unsafe, it was touch and go whether the State of Rhode Island, the prosecuting body, would proceed to a retrial. In January 1985 it decided to do so. When it did, Claus decided to retain the services of Thomas Puccio, one of America's best-known trial lawyers. At his first trial Claus had relied exclusively on local lawyers, one of whom joined the new defence team. In addition to Mr Puccio himself, this included two very bright young lawyers who had trained under Mr Dershowitz, who was at that time an academic and appellate lawyer rather than a trial advocate.

In the first trial both prosecution and defence had unthinkingly accepted that Sunny's comas that occurred around Christmas time in 1979 and 1980 were caused by exogenous insulin, and the case therefore revolved on who had injected her with it.

By the time of the second trial, Mr Puccio, having listened to the experts he called in to advise him, was positive that no one had given Sunny insulin and that her hypoglycaemia was due entirely to other causes, and that he could demonstrate this to the jury. In the first trial Dr George Cahill had given expert evidence to the effect that both comas had been insulin-induced and his evidence was virtually unchallenged; in the second, this opinion came under detailed scrutiny and was found to be wanting.

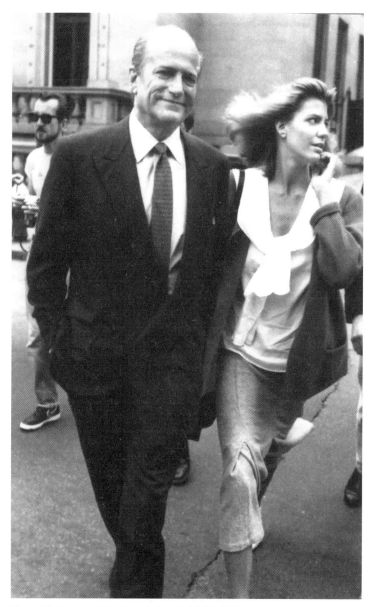

Figure 8 Claus and Cosima during his trial in 1985.

In preparation for the second trial Mr Puccio first approached Dr Harold Lebovitz, a distinguished New York clinician with an international record and expertise in diabetes and hypoglycaemia, for advice and help in assembling a group of independent experts who would review all the medical records – which ran to several hundreds of pages – from all the hospitals, and prepare reports. Mr Puccio decided that the experts should work independently of each other, disregarding what had been said at the first trial, the 'inquest' conducted by Mr Dershowitz that led to the appeal, and the media gossip of the past 3 years. This is where I came in, and it was probably an advantage that I had never heard of Claus von Bulow and could come to the court uncontaminated by the gossip and innuendo that had dogged the first trial. The other experts who agreed to testify at trial – once they had read the hospital records – included some of the biggest names in diabetes and hypoglycaemia research in America. They included Dr Arthur Rubenstein, Professor of Medicine at Chicago University, Dr Ralph DeFronzo, Associate Professor of Medicine at Yale University, Dr Daniel Foster, Professor of Internal Medicine at the University of Texas, and of course Dr Harold Lebovitz himself, Professor of Endocrinology and Diabetes at the State University of New York.

Mr Puccio also called Dr Leo Dal Cortivo, former President of the American Society of Forensic Toxicologists and Chief Toxicologist in the office of the Medical Examiner of Suffolk County, New York, and Dr Kurt Dubowski, a distinguished toxicologist and undoubtedly one of the world authorities on alcohol measurement and its interpretation.

Dr Dal Cortivo gave evidence about a hypodermic needle that the court had been told was found in Claus's black bag. The needle was described as having an encrustation on its surface that two prosecution witnesses had testified tested positive for insulin. Dr Dal Cortivo said that a hypodermic needle that had been used to make an injection would never have incrustations on its outer surfaces after it had been removed from the body. The conclusion that it had been tampered with seemed inescapable.

Although I had never met him, I was well acquainted with Dr Dubowski's work and often cited it, as I still do whenever I write anything to do with alcohol in a forensic context. He was the second of Puccio's expert witnesses to be called. He was adamant that the alcohol measured in Sunny's blood on the morning/afternoon of her admission to Newport Hospital on the 21st December 1980 was not an error even though its concentration would have been too low to have legal significance in a drink-driving case. Consequently it would not ordinarily be reported as positive. He was nevertheless emphatic that the concentration found at midday after several hours of total abstention was proof that Sunny had drunk a very substantial amount of alcohol the night before, whatever had been said to the contrary by prosecution witnesses. The amount of alcohol present allowed him to do a "back-calculation" of what she might have drunk on the previous evening. He pointed out that had there been absolutely no alcohol present, he would not have been able to conduct such a calculation. He considered it essential therefore to satisfy himself that the figure, though low, was genuine and not due to poor-quality analysis. He did this by examining the original laboratory records. He established that when the laboratory received a specimen that really did not contain alcohol, it reported a zero concentration. Only when alcohol was present did it report a figure. This may seem obvious, but it establishes the reliability of the laboratory process and is therefore an essential part of the forensic process. By doing this, he demonstrated that the report of an alcohol concentration of 9 mg/100 ml (2.2 mmol/L) was genuine even though, he admitted, the method used to measure it, an enzymatic technique, was not ideal.

Dr Dubowski explained to the court that since alcohol is not made in the body it must have got there by having been consumed. Moreover, it is accepted throughout the world that it is possible, providing alcohol is present in the blood – but not if it is absent – to extrapolate backwards to determine the least amount of alcohol that must have been drunk to produce the result obtained in the laboratory. Back-calculations, as they are called, are regularly used in drink-driving cases and assume that the average person destroys about 8 g of alcohol/hour by converting it to carbon dioxide and water. This produces a fall in blood alcohol concentration of about 15 mg/hour for men and 18 mg/hour for women. Providing the interval between ceasing to drink and measuring the blood alcohol concentration is known, it is relatively simple to estimate, within broad limits to allow for individual variations in alcohol metabolism, how much must have been drunk.

Dr Dubowski estimated, using a conservative figure of only 6 mg/100 ml/hour – or about a third of the expected rate for the disappearance of alcohol from the blood – that Sunny must have drunk at least 24–45 g (3–5 units) of alcohol before she went to bed. He considered it better to underestimate the amount required to produce the blood alcohol level of 9 mg/100 ml, measured around midday on 21st December 1980, than risk being accused of overestimating it. This level represents the amount of alcohol in 80–150 ml (3–6 units) of Scotch whisky: a more likely figure would have been at least three times as great, that is about 60–130 g of alcohol. This is equivalent to a quarter to a half a bottle of whisky, gin or vodka.

Mr Henry Gemma, the prosecuting lawyer, tried desperately to get Dr Dubowski to extrapolate back from the zero reading for alcohol found in

Sunny's blood on her first admission to Newport Hospital in 1979. He failed. Dr Dubowski did, however, point out that even with a zero reading it would have been quite possible for Sunny to have drunk quite a lot on the night of 26th December 1979, but he was of course unable to say whether she did or not. Mr Gemma also raised with Dr Dubowski the hoary old chestnut of the body as an auto-brewery. This story, which raises its ugly head every so often in drink-driving cases, postulates that the body sometimes produces alcohol within the intestine in exactly the same way as a brewery does by fermentation of sugars. Whilst this may be true to a miniscule extent, the idea that it ever does, or even can, produce sufficient alcohol to cause intoxication or more than an infinitesimal amount of alcohol in the blood is a myth. However, unless challenged by someone with real knowledge of the subject, the idea is sometimes put to and accepted by juries, leading to an acquittal on drink-driving charges. In Sunny's case Mr Gemma urgently needed to find some explanation for the alcohol found in her blood during her second coma, as he anticipated that I would say that alcohol was what had caused the hypoglycaemia and the coma.

Dr Dubowski was also quizzed, as was Dr Dal Cortivo, about the barbiturates that were found in Sunny's blood when she was admitted to hospital. The lab report had said she had a concentration of 10.6 mg/L of amobarbital in her blood, which, though generally not fatal, showed that she had taken considerably more than the standard dose for insomnia when she retired to bed on 20th December 1980. Dr Dubowski and Dr Dal Cortivo pointed out that although the report said amobarbital, the method of analysis used was incapable of distinguishing between the different barbiturates, and the substance was probably secobarbital (Seconal), another barbiturate with similar actions to amorbarbital. Sunny had been prescribed Seconal, along with Amytal (amobarbital), for many years by Dr Stock, her family doctor, to aid her sleeping. Its presence in her blood would have made her unsteady on her feet when she went into the bathroom on that fateful morning and slumped to the floor, possibly bumping her head on the way down. Her blood glucose, which was low at midday when measured in hospital, was probably sufficient to allow her to stagger from her bed to the bathroom, but too low to allow her to get up after she had fallen.

Dr Dubowski confirmed the testimony given earlier in the trial by Dr Dal Cortivo that Sunny must deliberately have taken some 60–65 aspirin tablets or more on the night of 1st December 1980 to give her a plasma salicylate level of 90 mg/100 ml on admission to Lennox Hill Hospital the following day. The prosecution lawyers and Dr Stock suggested that the high blood salicylate level could have been achieved by simple accumulation in the body from regular and heavy therapeutic usage. Anyone who knew anything about the subject would have dismissed this as nonsense.

After Dr Dubowski, I was the next witness to be called by the defence. This was not a logical sequence, but was determined by my need to be in Vancouver the following day to give a talk at a conference on clinical chemistry. Mr Puccio agreed to call me to the witness stand the morning after my arrival in Providence from London. We met for the first time over dinner the previous evening when he brought me up to date on the trial.

Next morning after I had given a short, and necessarily incomplete, explanation to the court of what hypoglycaemia is and how it produces damage to the brain, Mr Puccio asked me to say what I thought had caused Sunny's two comas. I pointed out that the first coma was almost certainly due to lack of oxygen to the brain and that the hypoglycaemia that she undoubtedly experienced was a secondary finding and not the cause of her coma. This opinion was arrived at independently of any of the other witnesses and it was only much later that I learned it was exactly the conclusion Dr Gailitis had himself reached and expressed to the court when he gave evidence for the prosecution.

I had read Sunny's medical records carefully, and the picture that emerged from them was totally unlike that of insulin-induced hypoglycaemia. In the first coma she had been blue and not pale or flushed, her blood was acidic and she was vomiting, all of which made me suspect from the beginning that insulin was not involved. My opinion was strengthened by the fact that Sunny took several days to recover completely after her blood glucose level was restored to normal. This suggested that her primary illness was an ongoing one, possibly an infection of her upper respiratory tract and lungs, made worse by inhaling vomit. This would account for her breathlessness during the afternoon and her blue appearance that Dr Gailitis noted when he was called to her home. It would also account for the vomiting, which is almost unheard of when insulin is the cause of hypoglycaemia, as Dr Foster was later to testify. It was not sufficiently appreciated in 1980, as it is now, that hypoglycaemia can result both from severe oxygen shortage and from infection.

As for the second and final hypoglycaemic coma, I had no doubt that this was due to a condition known as alcohol-induced fasting hypoglycaemia, and told the court so. This came as a surprise to many of the people in the court, because the public at large does not appreciate that alcohol can cause hypoglycaemia. Actually alcohol-induced fasting hypoglycaemia is much more dangerous to the brain than insulin-induced hypoglycaemia and is associated with a greater risk of death.

I based my conclusion entirely upon the objective laboratory data. The combination of alcohol and acidity in blood is typical of alcohol-induced – and unlike that of insulin-induced – hypoglycaemia. I did of course know that some alcohol had been found in Sunny's blood when she had been admitted to hospital and had independently arrived at the same conclusion as Dr Dubowski about the amount she must have drunk. I had also noticed from her clinical notes that Sunny consistently had large red blood cells during the whole of the year between comas (and possibly before then, but there was no information to go on). The two most important diseases that cause large red blood cells, namely vitamin B_{12} and folic acid deficiencies, had been ruled out, leaving chronic alcohol use as the most likely explanation. However, most telling of all was that during the first 3 months of her extended coma in 1981, when she no longer had access to alcohol, her red blood cells reverted to normal size. This was entirely consistent with a history of regular high alcohol use though not, of course, proof of it.

The clinical notes contained various allusions to Sunny drinking more alcohol than was good for her, and Dr Stock admitted, when he gave evidence for the prosecution, that Claus had mentioned this to him several years earlier. Sunny, not altogether surprisingly, had denied drinking heavily or consistently and was supported in her denial by her

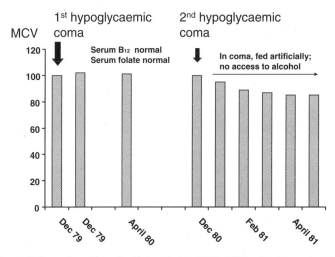

Figure 9 Sunny's red blood cell size during 1979–1981, showing restoration to normal after institution of artificial feeding and abstention from alcohol. MCV, mean red blood cell volume (in fL = 10^{-15})

two older children, her maid and her doctor, which is also not at all unusual.

There was convincing circumstantial evidence of Sunny's alcohol problems that was never exposed in court but that supports the medical evidence. After Claus's conviction at the first trial in 1982, over a dozen of Sunny's long-time friends came forward and volunteered sworn affidavits, which related to how often they had witnessed her totally incapacitated from drink over a period of many decades. These painful statements about a friend were filed as new evidence with the court between the trials but Mr Puccio did not consider it necessary to call their authors as witnesses. Moreover, unbeknownst to me and to Dr Dubowski, Alexander, Sunny's son, had already testified that on the evening of his mother's second coma he had carried her to bed before telling Claus, who had been in his study working for several hours, what he had done. This strongly suggests that Sunny was already the worse for alcohol by the time she went to bed and that her hypoglycaemic coma was alcohol-induced – after all, there is no other common explanation for an adult to be carried to bed.

The symptoms Sunny experienced when she was admitted to The Presbyterian Hospital for investigation of hypoglycaemia in the spring of 1980 were typical of alcoholic inebriation, although they can occur in other conditions, including hypoglycaemia, some serious neurological disorders and drug (including barbiturate) abuse. Hypoglycaemia due to an insulinoma was effectively ruled out and there was no objective evidence, either then or later, of any serious neurological disease. The question of alcohol abuse as a contributory cause of her illness was never pursued by the doctors treating her, because, as Dr Stock said, *"she denied it"*.

Sunny had been discharged from The Presbyterian Hospital with a diagnosis of reactive hypoglycaemia after the first coma. This is a more socially acceptable diagnosis than one of alcohol abuse. Alcohol abuse can, curiously enough, cause reactive hypoglycaemia in the course of a glucose tolerance test and the correct diagnosis can therefore be missed.

Like Dr Dubowski, whose evidence I had neither seen nor heard, I was quizzed about the significance of the alcohol reading of 9 mg/100 ml with, as I subsequently learned, exactly the same conclusion – namely that Sunny had drunk a considerable amount the night before her last coma.

Alcohol-induced hypoglycaemia generally comes on about 6–36 hours after drinking a moderate to large amount of alcohol. Something in the region of 50 g (6 units or 150 ml) of whisky is quite sufficient to produce it. Typically it occurs in people who are either malnourished or dieting and who have eaten very little food in the past 48 hours. It emerged during Dr Stock's cross-examination that Claus had specifically told him about Sunny's drinking in May 1976, when she had broken her hip. Interestingly, at the time of her hospitalization for aspirin poisoning in early December 1980, 3 weeks before her final coma, Dr Stock had described Sunny in the medical notes as being *"on a semi-starvation diet"*. There is no reason to believe that she did not continue on the same diet after her discharge. Dieting is of course exactly the condition that predisposes to alcohol-induced hypoglycaemia. It is also the most common type of hypoglycaemia to be associated with profound hypothermia because both alcohol and hypoglycaemia inhibit shivering, and shivering is the reason why most of us do not rapidly become hypothermic when we are exposed to the cold. There seems little doubt that Sunny was only scantily clad when she was found lying on the cold marble floor in her bathroom by Claus and her son when she failed to appear for breakfast. Even though the room itself was not unduly cold, it is not surprising that, with no shivering reflex, she had become hypothermic in the interval between about 6 am, when she was last seen in bed, and mid-morning when she was discovered unconscious.

The prosecution then turned to the plasma insulin results recorded by the commercial laboratory on the sample of blood collected soon after Sunny's arrival at Newport Hospital. They wanted to know how I could possibly ignore the very high insulin concentration of 216 mU/L (which is the way the laboratory reported the insulin concentration and is equivalent to 1548 pmol of insulin/L of blood) that the laboratory had reported on a sample of blood probably collected whilst Sunny was suffering from hypoglycaemia.

I agreed with the proposition that, if correct, the result would virtually have ruled out alcohol-induced hypoglycaemia as the cause of her coma since, had this been the case, both the insulin and C-peptide levels would have been suppressed to unrecordably low levels. As it was, her C-peptide level was either normal or low – depending on the sensitivity of the method that was used – but no one in the court seemed to want to know about C-peptide. I never did find out how reliable the C-peptide measurement was – especially as it was still a comparatively new test and the laboratory performing it was not one of the recognized reference centres. Nor did I learn exactly when the specimen of blood on which it was performed was collected. There was no evidence to show that the analysis for C-peptide was even done on the same sample as for insulin.

As for the insulin measurement itself, despite the importance given to it at the first trial, in which it had played a vital role in securing a conviction, there was good evidence that it was simply unreliable and wrong. The worthlessness of the result only came to light after the first trial was over. The sample of blood plasma on which the analysis was made had, as Dr Rubenstein would subsequently testify, been tested three times in two different laboratories with results of 0.8, 216 and 350 mU of insulin/L of blood; equivalent to 6, 1548 and 2520 pmol/L, respectively. No one – certainly none of the experts called by the defence – could accept such hugely divergent results as anything other than meaningless. It was, and still is, impossible to say which, if any, of the very different results was most accurate, and the range is so great that an average is as unreliable as the individual results.

Dr Cahill had relied heavily upon the figure of 216 mU/L (1548 pmol/L) when he had testified in the first trial that Sunny's second coma was insulin-induced. In the second trial, after his attention had been drawn to how the result had been obtained, he admitted that he could not trust it. Instead he relied on the fact that the amount of glucose Sunny needed to bring her round and restore her blood glucose to normal was much greater than he believed should have been necessary had she not been given insulin. Mr Puccio called Dr Ralph DeFronzo to refute this conclusion.

Dr DeFronzo is the person in the world who had done most to establish the relationship between insulin concentration in the blood and the rate of disappearance of infused glucose from it in healthy and sick people. Dr DeFronzo pointed out that, far from proving that Sunny's second coma was caused by insulin, the evidence, such as it was, argued very strongly against it. Had the blood insulin, level indeed been 216 mU/L (1548 pmol/L), she would have needed very much more glucose than she was given to raise her blood glucose from 1.6 mmol/L at noon when she was admitted to 14.5 mmol/L at 7.00 pm when it was next measured. Indeed, the amount she was actually given was just what he would have expected providing she had not been given exogenous insulin.

By the end of the trial the court had heard that not one of the experts called by the defence believed that insulin had anything to do with either the first or the second coma, and, as even Dr Cahill now had his reservations, the prosecution no longer had a case. The only dissenting voice was the evidence given by Dr Robert Bradley of Harvard University, who had testified for the prosecution that he was 100% sure that the first coma was due to exogenous insulin, and 99% sure that the second was.

The evidence of Sunny's maid, Maria Schrallhammer, so crucial in the first trial, was shown to be flawed, especially her claim that she had discovered a vial labelled insulin in Claus's black sponge bag. This was exposed in court to be, to put it politely, a mis-recollection and what others would have described in stronger language.

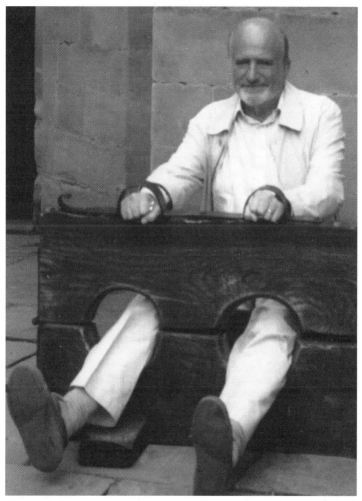

Figure 10 Claus playing up to his perception of himself as still in disgrace after his acquittal.

The jury were sent out to consider their verdict late in the morning of 7th June 1985, having heard evidence from some of the world's greatest authorities on hypoglycaemia. All of the experts believed that Sunny was the victim of natural illness and her lifestyle. In the first trial the main question had been who had given her the insulin that was supposed to have caused her hypoglycaemia on each of the two occasions. In the second trial this was not an issue. No matter how strong Claus's motivation may have been – and there was scant evidence of any – he could not possibly have been guilty of attempting to kill his wife, as no one had done so. And so the jury found when they returned their not-guilty verdict on the 10th June 1985.

After Claus's acquittal his stepchildren initiated civil litigation based on exactly the same evidence as had been rejected in the criminal case, no doubt on the basis that even if a jury could not be certain that Claus had tried to kill Sunny, a different jury, in a civil case, might still be gulled into thinking that he probably did so. Claus had, through his lawyers, already stipulated that he was prepared to divorce Sunny and waive any rights to her fortune providing the stepchildren were prepared to share the inheritance from their joint grandmother with their sibling, Cosima. They refused this offer for a further 3 years of civil litigation before finally agreeing to it.

The von Bulow case highlights how a prosecution case that is totally without merit and that should never have been initiated in the first place can lead to an innocent person being convicted of a non-existent crime, merely for lack of expert knowledge and the difficulty of conveying complex scientific facts to a judge and jury.

This was the first criminal case in which immunoassay played a vital role in elucidating the role of insulin in inducing hypoglycaemia and proved to be wanting. It illustrated the problems encountered in using methods and techniques that serve a useful purpose in clinical medicine but are not necessarily suitable for use in the forensic situation. This is a recurring theme throughout this book, in which at least one other miscarriage of justice was, in my opinion, based on misinterpretation of unreliable laboratory data (see the Winzar case, page 103).

It never ceases to surprise me when I meet people who know that I was involved in the case that many of them still believe from the stories they have read in the gossip sheets that Claus von Bulow was guilty but that clever lawyers had managed to get him off. The most prominent murder trial journalist in America at the time of Claus's trial was Dominick Dunne, whose reports of the trial, later incorporated in a book, are in no small way responsible for these misconceptions. He has left no one in any doubt where his own sympathies lie. In his book *Justice*, published in 2001, Dunne described how, whilst staying at Newport as the guest of Claus's stepchildren during the second trial, he came across *"a handsome box on his* [Claus's] *bed table"*. Dunne opened the box and under some cartridge shells *"was a used syringe"*, the significance of which is left to the reader's own imagination. As Claus had not been in the Newport house for several years, and since the crime scene bedroom had been carefully searched by the prosecution investigators on several occasions, this miraculous discovery, allegedly right in the middle of the second trial, was, not surprisingly, left unutilized by the prosecution, who declined even to disclose it to the defence attorneys.

There is little doubt that had Claus not had wealthy and influential friends who were prepared to lend him the money for his defence, he would not have received justice and would now be in prison for a crime that never was. Alan Dershowitz, who should know, reckons that Claus's various trials cost at least $3.5 million.

Claus now lives in London and is a well-known and highly regarded theatre critic for some of the better newspapers and literary magazines. Sunny survives in a vegetative state 25 years after the terrible illness that left her so brain-damaged that without constant attention she would undoubtedly have died.

5 Dolores Christina Miller, USA: why did she bother to kill a dying man?

Dolores Miller, a 52-year-old practice nurse, stood trial in Franklin County Court, Missouri, USA in February 1984 on the capital charge of killing her 10th husband, Erroll, also known as Roy, to whom she had been married for just 13 days before his admission to hospital for what proved to be an incurable brain tumour.

Erroll was a 59-year-old war veteran who, it later emerged, had developed fits and undergone a dramatic personality change some 2 months earlier. He had left a secure job and his family after withdrawing his life savings from the bank and before meeting Dolores through a lonely-hearts club. They lost no time in getting married, but as Erroll's symptoms got progressively worse he was admitted to the Harry Truman Veterans Hospital in Columbia, Missouri. There he was diagnosed as having a malignant brain tumour, for which he underwent brain surgery on 26th February 1983. The surgeons found it impossible to remove the entire tumour and his new wife was told exactly how serious his condition was. She was advised that that he was not expected to live very long – almost certainly less than 6 months.

Despite his continuing inability to speak, Erroll's recovery from surgery was uneventful until on the evening of the sixth postoperative day he became unconscious and had to be resuscitated. This happened while he was being taken to the X-ray department for a follow-up brain scan. Blood collected for routine analysis was found to have an unexpectedly low level of glucose. Upon hearing this result his doctors immediately gave him glucose intravenously, firstly as boluses but later by constant intravenous infusion. In all he required a massive 260 g of glucose over a 9–11-hour period before his blood glucose level was fully restored to normal. This was not accompanied by recovery of consciousness, and despite his blood glucose being normal he remained comatose and died 4 days later. Autopsy revealed only signs of persistent brain tumour and no evidence of an insulin-secreting tumour of the pancreas or any other cause for his death.

This was, however, far from the end of the story. From the day he was first found to have hypoglycaemia, Erroll's doctors suspected that it was caused by insulin someone had injected into him. The main suspect was inevitably his new wife, who was a nurse. From then on she was watched like a hawk whenever she visited her husband in hospital and was never left alone with Erroll in his room.

Dolores was visiting Erroll on the day he died. Shortly before his demise Dolores had collapsed over the intravenous infusion lines that were trailed across his bed while the nurse who was looking after him was adjusting his medication. As she flung herself over him Dolores had cried out that Erroll was dying but the nurse noticed nothing different about him. Shortly afterwards she observed on the cardiac monitor that he had developed an irregular heartbeat but, try as she might, she could not reverse it and he died shortly afterwards.

Blood collected just before his death was later assayed in the laboratory and found to contain no detectable glucose – in other words he had suffered another profound hypoglycaemic attack. A further sample of blood collected almost immediately after death also contained no measurable amounts of glucose. Plasma from these two blood samples together with plasma from blood collected before, during and after the original hypoglycaemic episode, and which had been retained in the laboratory refrigerator, was available for further analysis not only for its glucose but also for its insulin and C-peptide content.

Just as in the Claus von Bulow case, neither of these measurements could be done locally and the samples were sent to a commercial laboratory in California for immunoassay. The results did not become available until after Erroll's death but when they did they clinched the diagnosis of insulin-induced hypoglycaemia.

Dolores was already in police custody by the time of Erroll's autopsy, having been charged with driving without a valid licence. This made it easy for the local police detective investigating Erroll's death to confront her. This was done immediately it became evident that there was no anatomical cause for his hypoglycaemia, even before the results of the insulin assays had become available. The detective accused her of poisoning her husband with insulin, which was present in high concentration in samples of blood collected when he had his first hypoglycaemic attack. The absence of C-peptide from the same samples of blood established that the insulin source was pharmaceutical insulin and not Erroll's pancreas. Confronted in this way, she broke down and confessed, saying she had indeed given him insulin intravenously but not with the intention of killing him but solely to get him transferred back to the intensive care ward.

By the time the case came to trial, it emerged that Dolores had, prior to Errol's death, withdrawn all of her new husband's savings from the bank, wagered with hospital staff that he would be dead within a couple of days, and contacted several undertakers to find out how quickly a cremation could be arranged. Her car contained a stolen gun, lists of members of the lonely hearts club and several types of medicines and syringes – but no insulin.

At the time Erroll went into hospital many laboratories were able to measure insulin in blood but only a minority could also measure C-peptide. This is produced in the pancreas whenever it makes insulin and is stored along with the latter in the insulin-producing cells of the pancreas until they are both released into the bloodstream in response to the rise in blood glucose produced by eating a meal. Measurement of C-peptide along with insulin is useful in both clinical and forensic medicine as its presence in the blood helps to distinguish insulin made in the body from pharmaceutical insulin from a vial, which does not contain C-peptide.

By an amazing oversight, no insulin or C-peptide assays were ever carried out on the crucial blood samples collected around the time of Erroll's death when he had his second hypoglycaemic episode and from which he died. The hospital laboratory had shown that these samples contained no glucose, and this was considered by the doctors looking after him at the time and later by the prosecution as such incontrovertible evidence of insulin-induced hypoglycaemia that it was unnecessary to send the samples away for analysis. On reviewing the case to be presented in court the prosecution decided that the evidence linking Dolores with the second attack of hypoglycaemia was so weak that they decided not to introduce it. Everything therefore rested upon establishing that she was responsible for the first attack of hypoglycaemia and that it was caused by exogenous insulin.

The judge, however, ruled on legal grounds that certain crucial evidence relating to the insulin and C-peptide measurements made on the four samples of blood taken while Errol was suffering this earlier episode of hypoglycaemia was inadmissible. He did not question their accuracy or relevance – only that it was impossible to establish the chain of custody of the samples, which had been sent outside the confines of the hospital for analysis (that is to say, there was no direct evidence that the sample tested in the laboratory was the same sample, and in the same condition, as the one that had been taken in the hospital, even though, from an ordinary or clinical perspective, the sample was obviously the same one).

While this is perfectly acceptable in clinical practice, where to establish a chain of custody formally would make life virtually impossible for doctors and nurses looking after patients, it is an essential requirement in forensic work.

The immediate cause of Erroll's death was never ascertained. It was undoubtedly associated with and caused by his terminal hypoglycaemia. This was probably produced by insulin that Dolores injected into the intravenous infusion tubes when she sprawled over him on the bed on the last day of his life. The rapid fall in blood glucose that this produced would have led to the release of a large amount of adrenaline, which, in someone as ill as Erroll, could put a lethal strain on his heart. That is of course conjecture, since hypoglycaemia, no matter how severe, does not usually cause death unless it is continued for many hours or even days.

The fact that the results of the insulin and C-peptide analysis proving that Errol's hypoglycaemia was due to exogenous insulin rather than to some other illness were inadmissible as a matter of law reduced the prosecution's case against Dolores to little more than one of suspicion based on the strong circumstantial and clinical evidence and her confession (which she subsequently retracted). This was sufficient to convince the jury that Dolores had killed Erroll and was guilty of murder. She was sentenced to life imprisonment with a minimum of 50 years before eligibility for parole. The verdict was upheld a year later by the State of Missouri Court of Appeal.

6 Beverly Allitt, England: the nurse who killed babies

Beverly Allitt was the nurse who murdered at least four, and possibly more, small children in her care in Grantham, Lincolnshire, in 1991.

I was in Glasgow on 15th May 1991 chairing a meeting of the Association of Clinical Biochemists, of which I was at that time President, when I was called to the telephone urgently. All I was told before I got there was that it was the police. I had no idea what it was about and my anxiety level was high. My caller, who introduced himself as Superintendent Stuart Clifton of Grantham Police, quickly allayed my worst fears. The information department of NovoNordisk Ltd, a major pharmaceutical company and largest suppliers in the country of insulin for the treatment of people with diabetes, had given him my name. He was looking for someone who could help him measure insulin in blood and interpret the results. I replied that I could probably assist but that I was terribly busy just now and not quite sure when I would be able to help or even to meet him. We arranged to meet a week later in Grantham whilst I was on my way to Scarborough, where I was going to give a lecture on hypoglycaemia to the local medical society. Superintendent Clifton told me that he was investigating the possibility of multiple murders in Grantham Hospital and that insulin might have been used as the murder weapon – but they were still a long way off having a cast-iron case.

I arrived in Grantham and booked into the Angel and Royal Hotel, a wonderful old hostelry right in the centre of the town. About 6 pm Superintendent Clifton turned up – not alone, as I had expected – but together with three other men, including identical twins, both detective inspectors, who were part of his team of policemen and -women investigating what they believed to be one of the biggest multiple murder cases ever to have arisen in Britain.

It did not take long to establish that some of the cases they were interested in had been investigated in the very laboratory I had set up and developed in Guildford some 20 years earlier, mainly to investigate obscure causes of hypoglycaemia. Although I remained its official director, it was now under the day-to-day direction of Dr Derrick Teale.

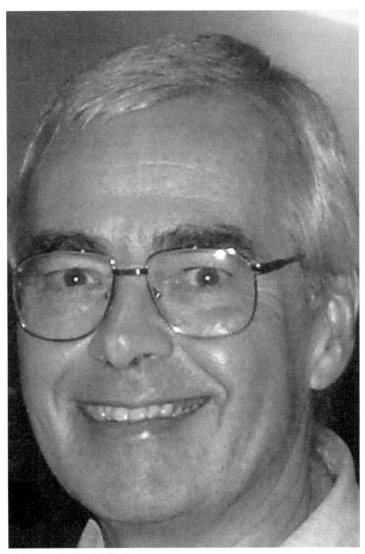

Figure 11 Dr Derrick Teale.

It turned out that although the police believed there had been serious wrongdoing in the paediatric ward – Ward 4 – at Grantham Hospital, and that although someone had been suspended on suspicion, the evidence was still far from conclusive. Everything that had happened, they had been advised, could have been due to an unhappy sequence of natural but tragic events.

The story they told me was fascinating but incomplete. I gave the assembled group some advice as to what further investigations needed to be carried out. These were mainly on specimens of blood plasma that had been collected from the various victims and which were being stored in refrigerators in Grantham and other nearby hospitals. Arrangements were made to deliver them to Dr Teale for analysis.

The results when they were obtained were dynamite. After they were communicated to Superintendent Clifton he was convinced he had a powerful case, but was less certain that all the experts he had consulted until then, mostly pathologists and paediatricians, would go along with him. He arranged to hold a conference to which all of them, and anyone else who had been involved in the case, were invited.

It was timed for early in the afternoon of Tuesday 2nd July 1991 and clashed with my outpatient clinic held at the Royal Surrey Hospital every Tuesday. Undeterred, Superintendent Clifton arranged for Surrey Police to collect me from the hospital at the end of my clinic and ferry me to Fair Oaks Airfield near Egham, about 20 miles away, from where I would be flown in a light aircraft to Cranfield, a similarly small airfield near Grantham. I remember the flight extremely well – rather better in fact than the conference itself. It was my first ever taken in a two-seater aeroplane and the pilot navigated by looking down at the countryside rather than by instruments; moreover the cockpit was open to the atmosphere.

The conference was attended by 60 or more people – about half of them from the police, with the remainder from various health institutions. There were 10 or so outside experts who were there to address one aspect or another of child health, a number of nurses and doctors who had been involved with the care of one or more of the children, and a phalanx of clerks, managers and administrators.

Superintendent Clifton introduced the subject that had first been brought to police attention on Tuesday 30th April. Two events prompted the call to police by the Grantham Hospital authorities. One was a meeting, in late April, of a group of junior doctors at the Queen's Medical Centre (QMC) in Nottingham who had become concerned at the large number of sick children they had received for specialist care from Grantham Hospital during the past 2 months. Whereas previously they had received two or three seriously ill children a year from Grantham, which used QMC Nottingham as its tertiary referral centre, more than twice that number had been referred in just the last 8 weeks. As a result they concluded that something was amiss in Grantham and communicated their fears to Professor, now Sir, David Hull, the Professor of Paediatrics. He informed the managers at Grantham of their concerns and implied that if they did not call the police, he would.

Similarly, some 11 days earlier, Dr Frederick Porter, one of the two paediatricians in Grantham, had expressed his concern. Consultant child care at Grantham was provided by two consultants, Dr Porter and Dr Charithananda Nanayakkara, each working independently and therefore not in quite as good a position to see the whole picture as the doctors in Nottingham were.

I learned from Superintendent Clifton that they had built up a case against Beverly Allitt, who was the only person connected with all of the 13 cases they suspected had been deliberately caused. The first hurdle they had to overcome, however, was establishing not who the criminal was, but whether there was any crime at all. Dr Porter was pretty sure there was – at least as far as baby Paul Crampton was concerned. Dr Nanayakkara, on the other hand, remained to be convinced that the hospital was suffering from anything more than a run of bad luck and poor facilities. This was a view shared by many of the other experts the police had consulted, because, individually, there was nothing specifically that pointed to illness from an unnatural cause. It appeared that almost no one except me was prepared at the beginning of the conference to stick their neck out and say that foul play had definitely been committed on Ward 4. I did this on the basis of our own findings in the case of baby Paul, who had been injected with a huge dose of insulin on three or more occasions.

Once the ice had been broken others joined in, and by about 5 pm the police knew they had a case – so it seems did the press, who had gathered in force outside the conference hall at the hospital. It was, however, not until 2 months later, on 3rd September, that Beverly Allitt was arrested on suspicion of murdering Becky Phillips, one of identical twin babies who were 6 weeks old. Even so the police had to let her go. Another 2 months elapsed before the evidence was sufficiently strong to charge her with murder. A lot of people put in a great deal of work between my conference with Superintendent Clifton in May and Beverly's arrest in November when she was charged with murder. But there was still more to be done.

I submitted the first of my many expert witness statements on 6th September 1991. It ran to 28 pages of typescript and dealt with just four of the 19 cases whose case notes had been delivered to my office for detailed analysis. The total amount of documentation occupied 7 feet of shelf space. The case notes on six patients were, after thorough examination, dismissed as being far too tenuously linked to any potential deliberate harm to warrant further investigation. The four cases I concentrated on, because I felt that they fell largely within my area of expertise, included Paul Crampton, who fortunately survived physically unscathed, and three of the children Beverly was finally convicted of murdering in May 1993.

Paul Crampton, aged 5 months

Paul's case provided the main evidence of wrongdoing in the first place. His case was unique in my experience, and I now know why. It was my first personal case of attempted or actual insulin murder. The cause of his hypoglycaemia was the deliberate administration of insulin on three separate occasions.

Paul was admitted to Grantham Hospital on 20th March 1991 with a history of coughing and wheezing. He was only 5 months old but had already suffered from chickenpox, which he contracted when he was only a fortnight old. On this occasion he seemed to be getting better from what turned out to be a mild chest infection and was scheduled for discharge after being seen by one of the consultant paediatricians on the morning of Saturday, 23rd March. Late that afternoon he was observed to be cold and clammy, and one of the nurses, who it later turned out was Beverly Allitt, suggested that he might be suffering from hypoglycaemia and proposed that a bedside blood glucose measurement should be made using a BM stix. This is a strip of paper impregnated with reagents that, when mixed with blood containing glucose, changes colour. This can be read by eye or, by combining it with a reader the size of a mobile telephone, used to measure the concentration of glucose on a tiny drop of blood from a finger prick in just a minute or two. The result was completely normal and reported in the notes as being 3.7 mmol/L.

Paul's deteriorating condition during the evening was put down to a recurrence of his chest infection. The duty doctor, whose name has unfortunately been lost to posterity, was called to see him an hour or so later. By this time Paul was in a pretty bad way. The doctor's notes record that Paul was sweating even though he had a body temperature of 36.7°C. For someone who has an infection, this is slightly subnormal (during an infection it would normally be expected to be over 37°C). The duty doctor nevertheless did a further BM stix test for blood glucose at 7.50 pm. This gave the very low reading of 1.5 mmol/L and led him, correctly, to diagnose Paul as suffering from hypoglycaemia. The cause was unknown but could possibly have been an infection and, on this basis, he began treatment with a broad-spectrum antibiotic. First and foremost, however, he treated the hypoglycaemia by giving Paul a feed of 100 ml of SMA, a human milk substitute, containing about 7 g of sugar, which Paul took with gusto.

The doctor also set up an intravenous glucose drip containing 5% glucose, which he changed to 10% glucose half an hour later. The infusion rate was adjusted to supply 1 g of glucose/hour – which is quite a lot for a baby of 5 months weighing just 6.7 kg. On this regimen Paul began to look much brighter and by 10 pm he was described as clinically much improved. His temperature was, however, still subnormal at 35 °C. This is quite common in patients with hypoglycaemia, and a repeat BM stix test confirmed that Paul's blood glucose level was still only 2.6 mmol/L despite the feed and the constant intravenous glucose infusion.

The rapid rate at which glucose was disappearing from Paul's blood was fairly good evidence that his hypoglycaemia was due to increased use of glucose by the tissues rather than to an inability of his liver to produce it. Although the concentration of insulin in his blood was not measured at this time, there can be little doubt that it would have been abnormally high.

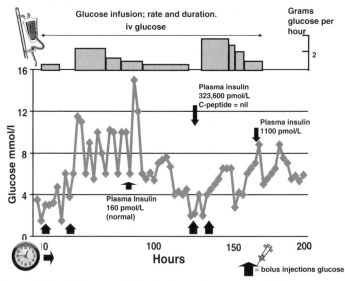

Figure 12 Paul Crampton's blood glucose levels during his hypoglycaemic episodes.

For the next 16 hours Paul continued to receive glucose intravenously and to take his regular feeds enthusiastically. A careful record of his blood glucose level was kept, using BM stix supplemented by laboratory tests on venous blood collected from time to time. By midday on 24th March Paul's blood glucose level was a very respectable 5 mmol/L.

The cause of the hypoglycaemia on this first occasion was most likely an injection of insulin into the skin or muscle and not intravenously, but it is impossible to be more precise. The injection was probably given an hour or so before the first real signs of hypoglycaemia appeared around 7.40 pm. This was more than 2 hours after Beverly had first suggested testing Paul for hypoglycaemia.

The dose of insulin used was probably not very large by adult standards – perhaps as little as 5 units – but this represents a large overdose in a 5-month-old baby. It was certainly sufficiently large to cause serious brain damage and possibly even death had the hypoglycaemia not been treated so promptly.

Paul's first episode of hypoglycaemia can be considered to have been over by early to mid-morning on Sunday 24th March. The glucose infusion was discontinued at 1 pm without any fall in his blood glucose level. By 2 pm the nurse's clinical notes report Paul as having *"become cold, clammy and drowsy again"* and his temperature had dropped to 35.5°C. A BM stix test at 2.20 pm gave a very low blood glucose reading of 1.0 mmol/L, which was confirmed by a laboratory test on venous blood collected at the same time. He was recommenced on intravenous glucose at a high dose of 3 g/hour. He was also given glucagon and cortisone therapy. By 3.00 pm he was more severely hypothermic with a temperature of 33°C, and his liver had increased in size. This was probably due to the accumulation of glycogen – the storage form of glucose made from the glucose he was receiving intravenously – under the influence of the large amounts of insulin in his blood. Liver enlargement is a feature of insulin poisoning in infants, and disappears almost as rapidly as it appears once all the insulin has been destroyed.

In addition to his ordinary feeds of SMA, Paul continued to need intravenous glucose for the next 4 days just to keep his blood glucose level within the normal range. During this critical period blood was collected and sent away for insulin assay. The result, which did not come back until after Paul had been transferred to QMC Nottingham, was reported as *"high normal"* but as the C-peptide was not measured on that sample it did nothing to solve the mystery of Paul's hypoglycaemia as it could have been a consequence of insulin made in his own pancreas.

With the benefit of hindsight there is little doubt that Beverly had injected Paul with a large dose of insulin at least 30 minutes before he developed hypoglycaemia for the second time at around 2.00 pm on 24th March 1991. The effect of this insulin continued for at least the next 2 days. It must therefore have been a long-acting insulin preparation given either into the skin or muscle.

Paul was still receiving intravenous glucose along with his normal feeds and he appeared to be comparatively well but still with residual evidence of the bronchial trouble that had brought him into hospital in the first place. In the early morning of 28th March 1991, 3½ days after the onset of the second hypoglycaemic episode, Paul's blood glucose was measured routinely and found to be rather low at 3.0 mmol/L. He was described in the clinical notes, however, as looking well and symptom-free. The intravenous glucose drip was still running but at the relatively slow rate of 10 ml, or 1 g, per hour, and by 9.00 am his blood sugar level was 5.0 mmol/L, which is well within the normal range. Even though he appeared now to have completely recovered from all his medical problems, the decision was made to keep the intravenous drip running for just a little bit longer – but very slowly.

Shortly after 1 pm one of the nurses on duty called a doctor urgently to the ward because the drip appeared to have become loose and to have leaked fluid into Paul's arm. He had also become very drowsy. A capillary blood glucose level was measured on the ward and had again fallen to hypoglycaemic levels.

The duty doctor managed to reconnect Paul's intravenous drip and to collect some venous blood for the laboratory before giving him a bolus injection of glucose and increasing his glucose infusion rate to 4 g/hour, which is a huge amount for a 5-month baby. The result from the laboratory confirmed the low blood glucose level and mentioned a low plasma potassium level. This was part of the routine measurements made and should have been normal – instead it was only 2.3 mmol/L. This is very low when compared with the lower limit of normal of 3.5 mmol/L and is commonly seen in patients with insulin-induced hypoglycaemia. Some of the plasma from this sample of blood was sent to a laboratory in Cardiff for insulin and C-peptide measurements, as these tests were too specialized to be done in the local laboratory.

Paul began to improve within 10 minutes of receiving the intravenous glucose and by 2.30 pm his blood glucose level was 4.0 mmol/L. By 3 pm he was wide awake and seemingly quite well. The decision had already been taken, however, to transfer him to the QMC Nottingham, where he could receive the specialist attention he clearly needed and which was beyond the capabilities and facilities of Grantham Hospital.

A bedside test for blood glucose carried out just before Paul was put in the ambulance to take him to Nottingham showed a glucose level of only 2.0 mmol/L. He was immediately given another bolus injection of 3 g of glucose before beginning his journey in the ambulance, which was made with the intravenous glucose infusion still running. The journey was uneventful and on Paul's arrival at QMC Nottingham yet more blood was collected for further tests. The glucose infusion was kept running at the very rapid rate of 40 ml (4 g)/hour for a further 24 hours and then gradually tailed off over the next day or so. The doctors looking after Paul still had nothing definite to go on as to what was causing his hypoglycaemia. It clearly had nothing to do with the infection that had taken him into hospital in the first place and had long since cleared up on antibiotic therapy. The doctors had not yet received the insulin and C-peptide results from the laboratory in Cardiff or the one in Nottingham itself, to which further plasma samples had been sent for analysis. This was not altogether surprising since insulin and C-peptide were not routine tests and still difficult to do. There was nothing to suggest that they were particularly urgent, as appropriate treatment for hypoglycaemia was already being given regardless of its ultimate cause.

Paul's recovery while he was in QMC Nottingham was uneventful and he was discharged fit and well on 4th March just 4 days after his arrival – but still without a definitive diagnosis, although malicious insulin administration seemed extremely likely.

Six other babies were admitted to QMC Nottingham from Grantham between 28th March and 22nd April, when the last of the babies attacked by Beverly Allitt died in Grantham Hospital. It was, as we have already said, this large and unexpected influx that led the junior medical staff at QMC Nottingham to approach Professor Hull with their suspicion of foul play at Grantham, the arrival of the police on the scene and Beverly's suspension from duty.

Claire Peck, aged 15 months

Claire Peck was 15 months old when she was re-admitted to Grantham Hospital on the afternoon of 22nd April 1991 suffering from "status asthmaticus". Her death, the last known to be caused by Beverly Allitt, also established the closest link with Beverly. Although it had nothing to do with insulin, Claire's story is included here as part of the overall picture and the part it played in bringing Beverly to justice.

Claire had been in the hospital several times since her birth and had been an inpatient only the week before with suspected asthma. Her final admission was because of suspected status asthmaticus, a life-threatening form of asthma in which the patient finds it increasingly difficult to breathe properly due to spasm and swelling of the tubes carrying air from the mouth to the lungs. The patient can neither get oxygen into nor carbon dioxide out of their body, and unless treated properly it can have a fatal outcome.

On admission to the emergency room of Ward 4 of Grantham Hospital a test of Claire's blood gases revealed that she was suffering from low-level carbon dioxide retention. This was an indication of the comparative mildness of her condition and not therefore a sign of status asthmaticus – but nevertheless an indication of the need for urgent treatment. She was seen first by a Dr Ratnayakara, a junior doctor who treated her with a salbutamol inhaler but with only limited success. He then inserted an intravenous cannula with the intention of treating Claire with aminophylline. This is an old but proven remedy for asthma that has to be given by intravenous injection very carefully and in a dose appropriate for the patient's weight. Claire was left in Beverly's care while Dr Ratnayakara went to see Dr Porter to determine and prepare the correct dose of aminophylline.

A few minutes after he had left, a more senior, but still student nurse, Nurse Sargeant, returned to the treatment room only to find Claire dark blue in colour and gasping for breath. Nurse Sargeant had left the treatment room just before Dr Ratnayakara in order to tell Claire's parents what was going on and had left Claire in Beverly's charge. Immediately she saw what was happening, Nurse Sargeant gave Claire oxygen through a mask, which led to her colour gradually returning to normal. By the time Dr Porter had got to the ward and seen Claire her colour was a normal pink and he proceeded to inject her with the aminophylline he had prepared. This took about 20 minutes or so and on its completion Claire appeared to be doing so well that she was being considered for discharge.

Once again she was left in Beverly's charge. An hour later Beverly raised the alarm. Claire, she said, had suddenly gone blue and stopped breathing. Nurse Sargeant and Dr Porter arrived moments later to find that Claire was no longer breathing and that her pulse was barely detectable before stopping completely. Dr Porter attempted to resuscitate Claire by external massage of the heart but could not get it going again. He did, however, collect some blood from her at 5.15 pm and sent it to the laboratory for analysis. Claire was still showing signs of life at the time the blood sample was collected and although she was breathing spontaneously her heart just would not start beating normally. After keeping up attempts to get her heart started, Claire was declared dead at about 8.15 pm. Dr Porter collected a further sample of blood from the right side of Claire's heart at 8.45 pm, about 30 minutes after her death. It was intended to analyse this at a later time to see if it would throw any light on her mysterious illness.

Mr Alan Wills, the laboratory technician on duty at Grantham Hospital, was summoned to return to the hospital and he arrived at about 9.00 pm. He commenced by carrying out an analysis on the blood collected from Claire just after she had died. He was astonished to find the concentration of potassium was so far above the normal range that his machine could not register it. So surprised was he, by this unexpected result that he confirmed it on another instrument elsewhere in the laboratory, and to reassure himself that the result was not due to contamination he examined the blood sample that had been collected while Claire was still alive. This too contained so much potassium that it was above the range that his machines could measure. Mr Wills issued a single result summarizing the two sets of results on plasma potassium as being *"in excess of 10.0 mmol/L"*. Fortunately he kept some of the plasma from each of the samples of blood collected from Claire before and after her death and put it into the deep freeze so that it could be analysed later if deemed necessary. Amongst the other substances Mr Wills measured at the time was Claire's blood glucose. This was very high, no less than 26 mmol/L, which is some five times the normal fasting level.

Until the police arrived on the scene nothing dramatic, apart from a mysterious fire in a mattress on Ward 4 on 29th April, seemed to happen at Grantham Hospital following Claire's death on 22nd April. Behind the scenes, however, the junior doctors at QMC Nottingham and Drs Porter and Nanayakkara at Grantham were all doing their bit to get the nursing and management authorities to take the escalating number of untoward events occurring in the hospital seriously. Eventually, on 30th April, the police were called in and on 1st May Superintendent Stuart Clifton visited the hospital for the first time. He recognized immediately the need for action and by examining the duty rosters identified Beverly as the prime suspect. She was suspended from duty.

This did not prevent her from seeking and obtaining other jobs both within and outside the NHS, where she continued to wreak havoc until she was arrested for the last time and kept in custody in November 1991. This was more than 9 months after the death of the first baby she murdered and 24 months before she was tried and found guilty of the murder of four children, the attempted murder of another three, including Paul Crampton, and inflicting grievous bodily harm on a further six children. She was also accused, after she left Grantham Hospital, of attempting to murder a 14-year-old boy, Jonathan Jobson, with the blood sugar-lowering drug glibenclamide, and an elderly inmate of a residential home, Mrs Dorothy Lowe, with insulin, but at her trial there was insufficient evidence to convict her on these charges.

Beverly Allitt insisted throughout her trial that she was innocent, but eventually, some months after her conviction when she was in Rampton Hospital, having received 13 life sentences, she admitted to Superintendent Clifton that she was responsible for three of the murders and six of the assaults. Superintendent Clifton has never revealed which of the 15 cases Allitt admitted to committing, as he thought it would be divisive and unnecessarily distressing to the parents.

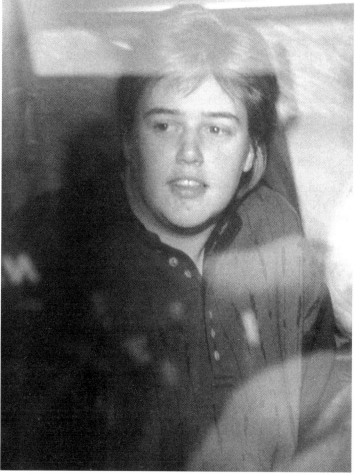

Figure 13 Beverly Allitt. Photograph reproduced with permission from Topham Picturepoint.

During the 24 months that elapsed between suspicion falling on Beverly Allitt and her coming to trial an enormous amount of effort was put in by the police and the experts they called to advise them. With the benefit of hindsight the whole scenario seems obvious, but it certainly was not at the time. It had to be demonstrated first that the events that took place on Ward 4 at Grantham Hospital could not have been due to natural causes and an unusual run of extremely bad luck, and secondly that if there really was foul play going on then only Beverly Allitt could be the culprit.

By the time I was consulted, the police had, by examining the nursing time sheets, established statistical evidence linking Beverly with each of the suspect hospital cases. There was a remarkable coincidence between the times when she was on duty and the occurrence of unexpected events in all 13 children. The chance of this being coincidence was calculated to be less than one in 10 million.

Nevertheless each child's illness could have had a perfectly natural explanation – apart from Paul Crampton's, Claire Peck's and Becky Phillips's – and even in their cases there was an extremely remote possibility that in each individual the damage was accidental. It was only when all the cases were taken together and had been investigated in greater detail than had originally been considered necessary for clinical purposes that the whole thing fell into place. It was this dotting of the i's and crossing of the t's that took so long.

Paul Crampton's hypoglycaemia was the first incident to be investigated with a rigour that could withstand scrutiny in the witness box. The blood sample that revealed what Beverly was up to was the one collected during Paul's third attack of hypoglycaemia on 28th March, before he was treated with intravenous glucose and sent off to QMC Nottingham. An earlier specimen, collected on 25th March and sent to the supraregional insulin assay laboratory at Hammersmith Hospital in London for analysis, had produced a normal result. This was scarcely surprising, since Paul's blood glucose level was normal at the time and so occasioned no comment from the laboratory. C-peptide was neither asked for nor measured on that specimen but would almost certainly have also been normal.

Paul's second plasma sample had been sent to the Supraregional Assay Laboratory in Cardiff, this time with a request for both insulin and C-peptide assay.

Dr Porter had, by the time of Paul's second episode of hypoglycaemia, become suspicious that Paul's hypoglycaemia might be due to a rare but very interesting abnormality of the pancreas that occurs almost exclusively in children. This condition, known as nesidioblastosis, produces an illness very similar to that of islet cell tumour or insulinoma in adults. It is characterized by hypoglycaemia produced by excessive release of both insulin and C-peptide from the patient's own pancreas. Diagnosis, once suspected, is pretty straightforward and seldom very urgent since the emergency treatment of hypoglycaemia is the same whatever its cause. It is characterized by the presence of high plasma insulin and C-peptide levels even when the blood glucose concentration is low. As described above, a high plasma C-peptide level serves to distinguish a pancreatic high insulin level from an equally high one produced by pharmaceutical insulin, which does not, of course, contain C-peptide.

March 29th and 1st April 1991 were Good Friday and Easter Monday, and so Paul's plasma sample did not arrive in Cardiff until 4th April. The sample was not dealt with until the next batch of tests was set up routinely on 12th April. By this time Paul had not only left Grantham Hospital but also QMC Nottingham, and was home with his parents. Dr Rhys John, who performed the assay, did not know this, however, and because the results were so abnormal he had phoned them through to Dr Porter in Grantham. The insulin level was so high that it went beyond the measuring scale used in Cardiff. The plasma C-peptide level, on the other hand, was so low that it could not be detected.

What then happened is described in some detail in the *Clothier Report*, the official report on the Beverly Allitt murders, which pointed out that Dr Porter, not being an expert on hypoglycaemia, had tried to get in touch with Dr Johnson, the paediatrician in Nottingham who had looked after Paul while he was in QMC Nottingham. Dr Johnson happened to be away and so was unable to help interpret the results. Even so, Dr Porter was suspicious that Paul's hypoglycaemic attacks might have been caused by deliberate or possibly accidental insulin administration rather than by nesidioblastosis. He communicated his misgivings to Mrs DM Onions, the nurse manager of Ward 4, who in turn communicated Dr Porter's misgivings about the plasma insulin and C-peptide results to the police, and this was how I became involved.

It transpired in late May, when I had my first meeting with Superintendent Clifton, that my former laboratory in Guildford had received two samples of blood plasma collected from Paul whilst he was still in QMC Nottingham. These had arrived on 10th May and been regarded as routine samples since there was nothing about them or the request form that accompanied them to suggest otherwise. They were analysed for their glucose, insulin and C-peptide content in the ordinary way. The blood glucose level in one of the samples was 4.5 mmol/L, insulin level 31 pmol/L and C-peptide level 439 pmol/L; and in the other these were 4.5 mmol/L, 28 pmol/L and 372 pmol/L, respectively, all of which were perfectly normal. The significance of these results only became apparent later when the results of tests carried out on samples of Paul's blood collected while he was suffering from hypoglycaemia on 28th March became available.

After my telephone conversation in Glasgow, Superintendent Clifton arranged for the remainder of the sample that had been sent to Cardiff and stored in their deep freeze to be collected and delivered to Dr Teale in Guildford. It arrived still deep-frozen in the capable hands of Detective Inspector Jones from Lincolnshire Police. The sample was duly analysed by a laboratory technician working under the direct supervision of Dr Teale who, like Dr Rhys John in Cardiff, found its insulin content to be so high that it was off the scale of measurement. Dr Teale did not stop here, however, but proceeded to measure insulin in carefully diluted samples of the original plasma specimen. The concentration in a sample that had been diluted 1 in 1600 was a staggering 207 pmol/L. This is equivalent to the astronomically high concentration of 331,200 pmol/L in the undiluted or original sample. He obtained similar results using smaller dilutions of 1 in 400 and 1 in 800 of the original sample, confirming that it really was insulin that was being measured and not just an artefact resulting from interference in the test procedure.

Dr Rhys John's results, which had already been reported, were so abnormal as to be outside anyone's experience in Grantham or in Nottingham. Consequently their accuracy and reliability had been viewed with some suspicion. Dr Teale's results not only confirmed but also extended them. Since both he and I, with our greater experience of such things, had seen similar results, we were not altogether surprised by them. They are almost always caused by insulin taken with suicidal intent and whilst we had never personally encountered a plasma insulin level quite as high as in Paul's case, Rosalyn Yalow, the Nobel Laureate who invented radioimmunoassay, had. She had found a similarly high plasma insulin level in an elderly woman who, it was believed, had been killed by an injection of insulin but for which no one was ever brought to trial.

Dr Teale, like Dr Rhys John in the Cardiff laboratory, could not detect any C-peptide in the sample of blood plasma collected whilst Paul was suffering from hypoglycaemia, nor could he detect any pro-insulin, the molecule from which insulin is made. Pro-insulin can usually be detected and measured in blood when the insulin concentration is very high due to its overproduction by the pancreas – but not when the insulin has come from a vial. It therefore acts as a double check on the significance of the absent C-peptide.

Dr Teale also looked for antibodies to insulin. These can sometimes occur in the blood and give rise to erroneously high insulin results. None was present in Paul's blood, so that the evidence that Paul had been given a huge dose of insulin was by now overwhelming, especially when combined with all the clinical evidence. It was now necessary to see whether any of the other children Beverly was thought to have damaged had been given insulin. None had been reported to have suffered from hypoglycaemia, and since it is only by lowering the blood glucose level sufficiently to produce brain damage that insulin ever produces harm it did not seem very likely. Nevertheless a search was initiated to find surviving samples of blood plasma taken from any of the children that would be suitable for insulin testing.

Becky and Katie Phillips, aged 8 weeks

The first sample to be received in Guildford from the Grantham children after the discovery of the very high levels of insulin in Paul Crampton's blood was from Becky Phillips. It had been collected soon after her arrival at Grantham Hospital on the morning of 5th April 1991 where she was certified dead, probably – it was thought at the time – from sudden infant death syndrome (SIDS). Becky was one of identical twins born prematurely 8 weeks earlier. Both she and her sister Katie had been cared for in Grantham Hospital intermittently since their birth. Becky had been in and out of hospital several times with a history of vomiting but nothing serious had been found to account for it. Her last admission was on 1st April for the same troubles as before. On this occasion she was kept in for 4 days, but once again no cause was found for her illness and she was discharged fit and well in the late afternoon of 4th April. In addition to Becky, her mother took home with her some feed made up in the ward to save her the trouble of making it up herself.

Becky first showed signs of being off-colour at about 6.30 pm, some 2½ hours after getting home from the hospital. According to her mother, Becky slept until about 6 pm, when she woke up unhappy but not hungry. She refused the food that she was offered and at about 7.30 pm she looked rather odd. Her eyes kept rolling about so that the whites showed. This lasted for only about 10 seconds and her mother put it down to colic. About 30 minutes later, just after 8.00 pm, Becky's father tried to comfort her and was successful in getting her to take 3 oz (approximately 85 ml) of feed. She would not settle, however, and at 10.15 pm her parents called their GP, Dr Higgins. He arrived at the house just 15 minutes later at 10.30 pm. He too diagnosed colic and suggested that Becky should be given some more food, which on this occasion she took avidly. After feeding, Becky seemed very much better and Dr Higgins left on another call saying he would return later – which he did. He examined Becky and found nothing wrong with her, and attributed the episode of eye rolling as due to colic. Becky was put back to bed and seemingly settled satisfactorily.

At 2.30 am, while Becky's twin sister was being fed, Becky woke up and began to grizzle. Her mother described her as crying, unsettled and sweaty. She took Becky into their bedroom and tried to feed her but she refused it. Soon after this Becky stopped breathing. Despite her parents' attempts at resuscitation, Becky failed to respond and she was rushed to the A&E Department* at Grantham Hospital, where, at 3.20 am, she was pronounced dead.

Dr Nanayakkara, whose patient Becky was, collected a sample of blood from her heart soon after she had died as he thought it might be useful in helping to find out the cause of SIDS, the condition from which he thought she had died. The blood was immediately separated into the red blood cells and serum, and the serum was stored in the deep freeze against the time when it would be used – presumably for virus studies – to investigate the cause of the illness. This act was very fortunate as the collection and storage method was ideal for subsequent insulin and C-peptide assays, even though, at the time, there was absolutely no reason to suspect that they would be anything but normal and would not ordinarily have been tested for.

Imagine Derrick Teale's surprise therefore when – more than 2 months after Becky had died from presumed SIDS – he found, exactly as in Paul Crampton's case, that Becky's blood contained so much insulin that it had to be diluted several hundreds of times in order to measure it. After diluting the blood serum 800 times to bring it into the optimum range for the method, Dr Teale concluded that the insulin concentration in Becky's undiluted blood must have been a staggering 72,000 pmol/L. Although not as high as the level found in Paul's blood, it was far above the levels ever found except after suicidal or homicidal insulin injection. Exactly as in Paul's case, serial dilutions confirmed that this really was insulin and not just an artefact produced by the assay method. The fact that there was neither C-peptide nor pro-insulin in the serum established that in this case too the insulin had come from a vial rather than from Becky's own pancreas.

Dr Teale also measured the glucose level in the sample of Becky's serum since this was routinely done on all samples submitted to the laboratory for insulin assay; without it, interpretation of the result can be extremely difficult. Paradoxically – but not altogether surprisingly – it was very high since, as had been established in the Kenneth Barlow case

---

* Emergency Room in America.

(see page 4), immediately after death glucose comes out of the liver and into the blood. Unless this fact is known and appreciated, it can cause confusion.

Much more difficult to explain than the high glucose level was the very high potassium level of 18.8 mmol/L that Dr Teale found. It has long been known, indeed ever since it became possible to measure it, that the potassium concentration in blood collected at autopsy is always higher than it was just before death. This is because as the cells of the body die the potassium they contain in high concentration during life leaks out into the blood. Even so, the concentration found in Becky's blood collected so very soon after her death was very much higher than could be accounted for by normal leakage. It is probable that Beverly had added potassium chloride to the feed she had prepared for Becky whilst she was in the hospital and which her mother took home with her. If so, it is likely that it was the potassium rather than hypoglycaemia that actually killed Becky.

As I pointed out at the trial, and Professor Edwin Gale for the defence emphasized, there was virtually nothing in her clinical history to suggest that Becky showed any of the classical features of hypoglycaemia during the 11 hours she survived following her discharge from hospital, where she must have been given the insulin injection, if indeed she was. The reason for this remains a mystery and, with the benefit of hindsight (see page 130), casts doubt on the validity of the insulin assay even though it was performed meticulously and to the highest standards using the methods prevailing in 1991.

The day after Becky's death, and long before the insulin assays described had been carried out, her twin sister Katie was admitted to Grantham Hospital, not because she was ill but as a precautionary measure. During the afternoon whilst being "specialled" by Beverly Allitt, Katie had stopped breathing but recovered quickly once a senior nurse arrived on the scene. The same thing happened the next day but this time she took longer to recover and started having fits. As soon as she had recovered sufficiently to be transferred, she was sent to QMC Nottingham for further investigation and treatment. Despite their best efforts, they found nothing to explain her illness and certainly no evidence of hypoglycaemia. Unfortunately she had already sustained permanent brain damage.

Superintendent Clifton was told the results of the insulin assays on Becky's blood on 18th June and this confirmed in his mind that they were dealing with a serial murderer – though the evidence as to who it was – was still far from complete. Inspector Jones, one of identical twin Inspectors Jones, was assigned the task of tracking down further specimens of serum remaining tucked away in deep freezers from other children who were suspected of being Beverly's victims. On 25th June he delivered samples from five of them to the Guildford laboratory, including some from Becky's twin Katie. Dr Teale diluted the samples as he was expecting to find high insulin levels. However, the insulin levels were normal. C-peptide levels were also normal, ruling out the possibility of malicious insulin levels.

Amongst the five samples was one collected from Claire Peck immediately after her death and containing evidence of the abnormally high concentration of potassium that killed her. Dr Porter had originally sent this sample to the Cardiff laboratory for insulin and C-peptide analysis on 25th April. Dr Rhys John had reported that, although it contained a large amount of insulin – 1175 pmol/L – it also contained substantial amounts of C-peptide (1000 pmol/L). This effectively ruled out the possibility that the insulin had come from an injection or that Claire had been suffering from hypoglycaemia immediately prior to her death. Dr Teale obtained an almost identical C-peptide result to that obtained in Cardiff but there wasn't enough blood for him to measure its insulin content.

A possible explanation for the high insulin and C-peptide levels in Claire's case was stimulation of insulin secretion by a combination of the aminophylline and salbutamol she had been given legitimately for her asthma. Both drugs are known to stimulate insulin secretion by the pancreas. Under some conditions intravenous potassium chloride – which Beverly had given her illicitly – can also do this and may have been a contributory factor.

A potential red-herring introduced into the cause of Claire's death was the finding of a drug, lidocaine, in the blood sample collected at 8.45 pm, half an hour after her death. Lidocaine is a local anaesthetic, which, in much larger doses, is used to correct irregularities of the heart beat. At the dose found, 5.8 μmol/L, it was just below the optimum concentration for use as a cardiac drug, but how it got into Claire's blood remained a mystery since Dr Porter had neither prescribed nor given it to her. In any event, it is extremely unlikely that it played any role in Claire's death. It nevertheless gave the lawyers something to think and argue about. Could Beverly Allitt have given it to her prior to the potassium chloride injection? This is the most likely explanation but impossible to prove. Someone else may have done it and forgotten that they had done so by the time of the trial more than a year after the event. The most likely explanation, however, is that the specimen containing lidocaine came from someone else. In other words, there was a mix-up somewhere between the collection of Claire's blood and the reporting of the lidocaine result. This is exactly the sort of problem the judge in the Dolores Miller case had in mind (see page 53) when he refused to permit the results of some laboratory test to be given in evidence.

Liam Taylor, aged 7 weeks, and other Allitt cases

Two other cases came to light in which insulin may have played a role between the time Beverly Allitt was suspended from Grantham Hospital and her arrest on charges of murder. In neither of them was the evidence of guilt sufficient to convince the jury and she was acquitted of both charges.

Beverly was, however, convicted of killing two other children in addition to Claire Peck and Becky Phillips, of attempting to murder three others – including Paul Crampton – and of causing grievous body harm to another six children on Ward 4 of Grantham Hospital.

Insulin could only be implicated in one of the other Grantham Hospital cases, and even here the evidence is indirect and not very convincing. Liam Taylor was 7 weeks old when he was admitted to Grantham hospital with a history of coughing, wheezing and sticky eyes on 21st February 1991. An X-ray of his chest revealed that he had pneumonia, for which he was immediately given antibiotics. Two days later, after an apparently uneventful recovery, he suddenly collapsed from what was described as a cardiorespiratory arrest at 4.13 am on 23rd February 1991. He did not respond to attempts at resuscitation, and died.

An autopsy conducted by Dr Fagin found, as almost the only abnormality, an enlarged liver stuffed full of glycogen, the storage form of glucose. Glycogen is made in the liver under the influence of insulin secreted in response to a meal, and is gradually broken down once the supply of insulin falls as all of the meal is absorbed. This breakdown of glycogen provides the brain with the glucose it needs to survive during periods of fasting. Excessive deposition of glycogen in the liver is consistent with Liam having been given insulin maliciously, but is far from proof of it. Nevertheless it is a matter of public record that enlargement of the liver, detected during life and caused by excessive glycogen deposition, was the sole reason that an unrelated case of proven malicious insulin administration to a baby first came to light. In that case, however, unlike in Liam's, the baby's plasma insulin level was measured and was high. In Liam's case there was no serum available to test. Thus, whilst it is possible that Liam's cardiorespiratory arrest was caused by insulin-induced hypoglycaemia, the evidence isn't there. No blood glucose measurements were ever made before Liam's life support machine was switched off. If insulin was involved, it would probably have been given intravenously to produce such a devastating effect so rapidly. This was feasible as Liam was being given a slow intravenous infusion of glucose, and if a bolus of insulin had been injected into the infusion, it would have produced a rapid fall in his plasma potassium concentration, and this in turn could have caused a cardiac arrest.

Exactly how Beverly harmed the children she was convicted of killing, attempting to kill or causing grievous bodily harm to will probably never now be known. Beverly, after an unsuccessful attempt at starving herself to death, has been in Rampton Mental Hospital since her conviction and is expected to remain there for the rest of her life. Meanwhile the damage she has done as probably the most notorious of child killers of modern times lives on. In 1999, 8 years after the terrible events in Grantham Hospital, it was announced that the Phillips family had been awarded around £2,000,000 damages to provide for Katie Phillips, Beckie's surviving twin, for the rest of her life. The health authority had, some 3 years earlier, in a landmark decision, agreed to compensate, for the psychological damage they had suffered, the 12 sets of parents of the children attacked by Beverly during her brief period as an assistant nurse on Ward 4 of Grantham Hospital.

7 Jane Wagstaffe, England: was it suicide?

Jane Wagstaffe was a 34-year-old divorcee living in Hereford, a small English country town. She was found dying in her bed by her landlord, David Walton*, at around 4 am on 6th August 1995. He called an ambulance as soon as he discovered her and said that he had gone into her room after being disturbed by what sounded like choking noises coming from there. He described her as being very short of breath, but by the time the ambulance arrived she had already stopped breathing. The ambulance crew decided that there was nothing more that they could do and called Jane's own doctor. He came immediately and certified her dead. He found nothing amiss in a cursory examination of her body and later said that there were no suspicious circumstances surrounding her death.

Because Jane's death was unexpected, her GP reported it to the coroner, who ordered a post-mortem examination. This was undertaken the next morning, 7th August 1995, at around 9 am.

The autopsy was carried out by Dr Frank McGinty, Consultant Pathologist at Hereford County Hospital, and revealed no anatomical cause for her death. The only anatomical finding was severe congestion of the lungs (technically called pulmonary oedema), which Dr McGinty interpreted, I am sure quite correctly, as associated with, rather than the cause of, her death. Her stomach showed evidence of mild inflammation or gastritis and contained some dark-coloured fluid of no diagnostic significance, and there were no external or internal signs of violence.

The story that emerged when police began their investigation into Jane's death was that she lived in a house together with David Walton and his partner, Jennifer Runn*. They both reported that Jane had an alcohol problem in so much as she was a *"heavy drinker"* although she had never been in trouble, either medically or with the law, from alcohol abuse. Her GP was treating her with the tranquillizer lorazepam for

---

* Not his/her real name.

anxiety. She appeared also to be taking an over-the-counter proprietary sleeping pill but physically she was in reasonably good health.

By the time Dr McGinty examined Jane's body, the police had already ascertained that David Walton's partner was a type 1 diabetic and kept insulin in her refrigerator at home. The possibility that this might have been related to Jane's death prompted Dr McGinty to collect some of her blood for later analysis in the laboratory. He also took some fluid, called vitreous humour, from one of her eyes, as this is widely but wrongly, believed to be a reliable guide to the blood glucose concentration at the time of death. The glucose concentration in the vitreous humour was 0.12 mmol/L (i.e. virtually zero), which, while very low for a living person, is not necessarily so in someone who has been dead for more than 24 hours.

Analysis of the post-mortem blood sample revealed an alcohol concentration of 111 mg/100 ml (24 mmol/L), which, though well above the legal limit for driving, is insufficient to kill anyone – especially somebody known to be a heavy drinker. It also contained an insignificant trace of paracetamol: 4 mg/L. Thus no real cause for her death was found by this more or less straightforward coroner's autopsy.

Dr McGinty believed that the very low concentration of glucose in Jane's vitreous humour was consistent with death from insulin poisoning, which it is, and he arranged for the remainder of the blood sample he had collected to be sent to my laboratory in Guildford for analysis.

On arrival the sample was immediately analysed for its insulin and C-peptide content by radioimmunoassay but not, on this occasion, for glucose as the result would have been worthless in blood collected so long after death. The results obtained revealed an extraordinarily high concentration of insulin – equivalent to about 125,000 pmol (17 units)/L – and an undetectably low C-peptide concentration.

If correct, these results could only be explained by concluding that Jane had died from an excessively large dose of insulin, which would have had to be given by injection. The police were advised of the results and in discussions with them I suggested that a further and even more thorough search of Jane's body for puncture sites and depots of unabsorbed insulin was necessary. If any suspicious sites were discovered, they, and similar sites not considered suspicious, would be excised and sent to Guildford and tested for insulin.

No injection sites were identified by careful visual re-examination of the body, but, using a mechanical device borrowed from the police in Birmingham, two suspicious areas were discovered. Dr McGinty removed them and a further 14 tissue samples of similar size from Jane's body and sent them to Guildford. The samples were identified only by number so that the analyses carried out on extracts of them were performed blind – in other words, the analyst did not know which, if any, of the samples were suspicious and which were not.

Dr Derrick Teale performed the analyses using an immunoassay technique he had adapted from the one he used to measure insulin in blood. It was therefore many hundreds of times more sensitive than the methods used by Dr Gurd and Professor Pfeiffer in the Kenneth Barlow (see page 3) and Herr Breslau (see page 7) cases, respectively.

Only one of the 16 samples – the one obtained from the right hip region – contained substantial amounts of insulin. Many of the others contained miniscule but measurable amounts that could easily be explained by the high concentration of insulin in the blood they contained. The amount of insulin in the sample from the right hip was, however, far greater than could be explained in this way and must therefore have been due to residual insulin from an injection. The right hip was a place where Jane could easily have injected herself. The question now was did she inject herself or did someone else do it?

The police continued their enquiries, but only one more medical fact emerged to help, or possibly hinder, the coroner and his court to arrive at a cause for her death. Post-mortem examination had revealed that on the night of her death Jane Wagstaffe had had sexual intercourse. When questioned about this, David Walton admitted that he and Jane had consensual sex that evening. Although there was some evidence that on previous occasions Jane had rebuffed his sexual advances, there was nothing to suggest that she had been coerced into accepting them on this occasion.

In due course the coroner's jury returned an open verdict. Neither Dr Teale nor I were called to give evidence, since we had little to offer beyond what we had already reported. Clearly Jane had received a massive injection of insulin sometime during the previous late evening or night and it had either caused her death or contributed to it.

It was impossible, on the evidence, to say who administered the insulin. Although suspicion had originally centred on David Walton, the most likely person was undoubtedly Jane herself. There is no earthly reason why Jane would have let someone inject her with the 10–30 ml of insulin necessary to produce the sort of plasma insulin levels found in her body and yet not call for help in the 20 minutes or so that remained before she became unconscious from hypoglycaemia.

If Jane did inject herself, she must have disposed of the syringes, needles and vials of insulin that she used, as none were found in her room. She would have had plenty of time to do so before she succumbed to its hypoglycaemic effects. Her motives for taking her own life, if that is what she did, are anybody's guess. She did not leave a suicide note – but then many suicides do not. Suicide is common in heavy drinkers.

The rapidity of her death from hypoglycaemia (6–8 hours at the very most) is unusual, but may have been due to the combination of hypoglycaemia and alcohol, which is far more lethal than hypoglycaemia alone. If, as seems likely, she died around 6 hours after going to her bed, her blood alcohol level when she retired would have been much higher than the 110 mg/100 ml found in her body at post-mortem. I calculate, exactly as Dr Dubowski did in the Claus von Bulow case (see page 41), that when she went to bed, 6 or so hours before her death, Jane's blood alcohol concentration was in the region of 200 mg/100 ml, or the equivalent of about half a bottle of whisky. It is probably around this time, 6 hours before she was found dying, that the insulin injection was given.

It is very unlikely that we will ever know the true reason why Jane Wagstaffe died, though the cause is not seriously in doubt. The presence of insulin in the house and the insulin assay result indicating the presence of a large amount of insulin in her body both point in the same direction. The absence of C-peptide from the post-mortem blood sample and the finding of a depot of insulin in one of the tissue sites confirm that it was pharmaceutical and not endogenous insulin that killed her

But why, if it was suicide, did she do it? Was it anything to do with her recent sexual exploits and would this explain why she disposed of the evidence in the shape of syringes, needles and vials of insulin so that her death would be surrounded by mystery. Unless something extraordinary happens, the answers to these question will forever remain unknown.

8 Maria Whiston, England: the "insulin between the toes" case

Eric Lloyd had been in a relationship with Maria Whiston, a trained nurse who had come to Britain from the Philippines, from about 1990 up to the time of his death, 4 years later, at the age of 60.

Eric had not enjoyed very good health for some years and had last seen his doctor on 13th May 1994 (only 3 weeks before his death), when he was described as being generally low in spirits, his brother having recently committed suicide in America. Eric was currently living with Maria, whom he intended to marry. He had been married twice before. The first time was when he was 25. That marriage had lasted 14 years and gave rise to one daughter. The second lasted only 2 months and there had been no further contact with that wife since the divorce.

Although there were no particularly suspicious circumstances surrounding the death, the coroner ordered an inquest because it was both sudden and unexpected and, in the UK, it is a legal requirement if the deceased has not consulted their doctor in the preceding fortnight. The inquest was arranged for 5 days later, on Wednesday 8th June. Maria told the coroner that she had found Eric dead in bed on Friday morning 3rd June, when she returned from night duty at the hospital where she worked. She had called the family doctor, who came round to the house, certified the death and notified the police because Eric's demise was both sudden and unexpected. In the course of the inquest Eric's daughter, Karen, expressed concern about her father's death and made certain allegations against Maria. As a result the inquest was adjourned and the police began enquiries that eventually led to Maria facing a murder charge in Birmingham Crown Court on 4th June 1996, almost exactly 2 years after Eric's death. Even then, the trial was adjourned at the request of the prosecution, after they learned that the defence intended not only to question the accuracy but also the interpretation of the results of the insulin assays that had been undertaken on Eric's urine and which were absolutely crucial to their case. They asked for time to undertake more research.

PC Stephanie Stephens was one of the police officers who attended the scene, having been called to Eric's house by his doctor, who had not expected him to die so suddenly. She described Eric as lying on his bed with vomit on both sides and on the carpet. This led her to conclude that she was dealing with an unnatural death.

Later, after Karen's intervention at the inquest, PC Stephens said that the condition in which she found Eric's body seemed suspicious to her and consequently she had inspected the room and rest of the house more thoroughly than she otherwise might have done.

This revealed a number of items she thought worth recording. Amongst those she listed were two packets of paracetamol tablets from which 11 tablets were missing, another box of 50 paracetamol tablets, two packs of atenolol blood pressure tablets, similar to the propranolol prescribed for Sunny von Bulow (see page 33), from which 13 were missing, and a pack of Prothieden (dosalepin) tablets (an antidepressant) from which none was missing. She also found two pre-injection swabs on the window ledge. Doctors and nurses use these swabs, which are small pieces of cloth soaked in alcohol packaged in aluminium foil, to clean the skin before giving someone an injection – they would not ordinarily be found at someone's home. Having completed her inspection PC Stevens arranged for Eric's body to be taken to the public mortuary.

Professor Edward Lynn Jones, Professor of Histopathology at Birmingham University, made a post-mortem examination at 2.30 pm on 3rd June, less than 5 hours after Eric's death had been reported. In his mind was the possibility that he might have died from self-poisoning – in other words, that he had intended harming or killing himself.

Professor Jones found no obvious cause for Eric's death and no evidence of inhaled vomit, although he searched for it. There was mild bruising of the right thigh. Professor Jones recorded that Eric's heart was *"moderately enlarged due to ventricular hypertrophy"* and that the *"coronary arteries showed partial occlusive atherosclerosis"*. In other words, Eric had hardening of the arteries, which had caused approximately 50% narrowing of one of the large arteries going to the heart.

Because of the suspicion of self-poisoning, Professor Jones collected samples of blood, urine and stomach contents for analysis later in the laboratory, and pieces of the liver for histological examination. Everything was set up for the formal inquest, at which death from natural causes would, in all probability, have been recorded but for Karen Lloyd's intervention.

Dr Peter Acland, a Home Office Forensic Pathologist and Lecturer in Pathology at Birmingham University, carried out a second post-mortem examination immediately after Karen's intervention, on the afternoon of 8th June 1994. Dr Acland was told about two factitious (artificially induced) hypoglycaemic episodes that Eric had suffered a couple of years before his death. When added to the information that had already been given to Professor Jones and the concerns imparted to the coroner by Karen, he had good reason for suspicion that all was not quite what it seemed to be.

Dr Acland's post-mortem was no more informative, however, as to the cause of Eric's death but it did confirm the abnormalities of the heart and its blood vessels that Professor Jones had found. Despite meticulously and very deliberately searching for needle puncture marks that might indicate an insulin injection site, he found none. Nevertheless he took some of the bruised tissue from the right thigh – just in case it might be the site of an insulin injection – and a similar piece from the left thigh for comparison. He also collected a further sample of urine, some bile from the gall bladder and vitreous humour from both eyes (all now some 5 days old) for analysis in the Home Office Forensic Science Laboratory at Chorley in Lancashire. He was adamant, at a later time, that he had not collected any further blood samples – presumably because he knew that any information they might have contained could be elicited more reliably by analysis of the fresher samples collected by Professor Jones.

The factitious hypoglycaemic episodes of 1991

The history of factitious hypoglycaemia to which Dr Acland's attention had been drawn was as follows. On 26th August 1991, 3 years before his death, Eric arrived unconscious at the A&E Department[*] of East Birmingham Hospital. A routine blood glucose test, undertaken on everyone arriving in a coma, revealed that he was suffering from hypoglycaemia but the cause was unknown since he did not suffer from diabetes and had never been prescribed insulin. He came round immediately he was given an intravenous glucose injection but was unable to throw any light on the cause of his hypoglycaemia. He was admitted to hospital for investigation but no cause for it was found, and 4 days later, on 30th August, he was considered fit for discharge without a firm diagnosis.

He was readmitted via the A&E Department – less than 2 months later – on 22nd September 1991, again in a coma with a history, on this occasion, from Maria, that he had woken up with a headache and

[*]   Emergency Room in America.

vomiting. He had, she said, gradually lost consciousness during the course of the morning and was comatose by the time of his admission to hospital. The A&E Department again did an on-the-spot glucose test on capillary blood from a finger prick. This showed that he was suffering from hypoglycaemia and explained his coma. A further sample of blood, this time from a vein, was collected before he was brought round with intravenous glucose. The plasma from this blood sample was subsequently sent to Guildford, where it was analysed for glucose, insulin and C-peptide by Dr Derrick Teale. The results were not crucial to Eric's immediate treatment and consequently were not given priority and did not become available for several days.

Meanwhile, as before, Eric rapidly regained consciousness following a shot of intravenous glucose and was unable, as on the previous occasion, to throw any light on what had caused his coma. The blood glucose concentration in the venous sample collected in the A&E Department was only 1.3 mmol/L (it is normally between 3.5 and 7 mmol/L in the non-fed person, and still higher after a meal) and was sufficiently low to account for his coma.

During this hospital stay Eric's blood glucose level was measured at frequent intervals for several days. It fell below 2.5 mmol/L on some occasions in spite of the glucose he was receiving intravenously for much of the time, suggesting either the presence of an insulin-secreting tumour of the pancreas or a very large and certainly not accidental overdose of insulin from out of a bottle.

While the results of the insulin and C-peptide assays were awaited from Guildford and the cause of his hypoglycaemia was therefore unknown, Eric underwent further investigations in Birmingham, but again no cause was found. On the assumption that he must have been suffering from some form of endogenous over-production of insulin, due perhaps to an insulin-secreting tumour, he was treated with a drug called octreotide. This specifically blocks the secretion of insulin by the pancreas and is often used to treat hypoglycaemia arising from this cause. It has no effect on other types of hypoglycaemia, and had no effect in Eric, making an insulin-secreting tumour as a cause for his hypoglycaemia unlikely but still possible.

The sample of blood collected at the time of Eric's second admission to the A&E Department in Birmingham, and before the intravenous glucose injection, had an insulin content of 1576 pmol/L, which is high in absolute terms and quite inappropriately so for someone suffering from hypoglycaemia due to natural causes, when it is ordinarily undetectable, unless the patient has an insulin-secreting tumour of the pancreas. This was ruled out, however, by the fact that the concentration of C-peptide in the same plasma sample was undetectably low, that is it was less than 75 pmol/L. These results were communicated to Birmingham with the comment that they were consistent with a history of insulin administration and indeed were very suggestive of it. This was construed as evidence that someone had injected Eric with insulin on this second occasion and, by implication, on the first occasion, too. Far and away the most likely cause of this is self-injection of insulin giving rise to the well-recognized clinical condition of factitious insulin-induced hypoglycaemia. This is thought to be an attention-seeking device and must be distinguished from suicidal and the very rare homicidal use of insulin, in which much larger doses of insulin are generally employed.

Dr Teale did not test to see whether there was any pro-insulin present – pro-insulin is the molecule from which insulin is made in the pancreas – nor did he examine the blood sample for the presence of insulin antibodies as it was not relevant at the time – though it became so later after Eric's death and Maria's arraignment for his murder.

Insulin antibodies can, under exceptional circumstances, be a cause of hypoglycaemia as well as interfering with the measurement of insulin by immunoassay. They must therefore always be considered whenever there is any doubt about the cause of a patient's hypoglycaemia. This had not been an issue when Eric was ill in 1991, though it became so after his unexplained death in 1994.

Once the results from Guildford became available to Eric's doctors they confronted him with the fact that there was no explanation for his hypoglycaemia other than insulin injections, but he vehemently denied that he had ever been injected with insulin either by himself or anyone else. He persisted in his denial even to the psychiatrist to whom he had been referred and who was especially skilled in the art of interviewing potentially suicidal patients and those with injuries self-inflicted in order to gain medical attention and sympathy.

It was recorded in his hospital case notes that during his stay in hospital, immediately after the second hypoglycaemic attack, Eric was so concerned about being on the third floor that he requested to be moved to the ground floor. This behaviour is consistent with suicidal thinking and possibly relevant to subsequent events, but it was never discussed or explained either at the time or later.

Nothing of clinical significance happened to Eric over the next 2 years except that he did agree to go into hospital under the care of the consultant psychiatrist, Dr White, from 7th January until 13th April 1992. Yet again, not surprisingly, he denied ever giving himself insulin or, more significantly, letting anyone else do so. The last observation of possible relevance to what subsequently happened was the note made by his GP on 13th May 1994 that Eric was *"generally low in spirits, as his brother had committed suicide in America"*.

Less than 1 month after this note was made, Eric was found dead in bed. Was it death from natural causes, suicide or murder? The autopsy did not reveal an obvious anatomical cause and, after Karen Lloyd's intervention at the inquest, everything depended on the results of the toxicology examinations.

Toxicology results

The samples of blood, urine and vitreous humour collected at post-mortem by Professor Jones and Dr Acland were delivered, by hand, to the Home Office Forensic Science Laboratory at Chorley in Lancashire on 9th June 1994. They were examined by Dr Philip Owen, who carried out a limited range of drug analyses on the various samples. He found evidence of carbamezapine (a drug used to control epilepsy), thioridazine (a drug used to treat schizophrenia) and low levels of temazepam (a drug used to induce sleep) in the urine and blood – but no alcohol.

The stomach contained the equivalent of a tiny fraction of a tablet of thioridazine, but as the amount was so small, it had presumably not been taken in overdose. It also contained traces of an unspecified tranquillizer of the benzodiazepine group. Much of the stomach contents had been vomited onto the carpet and was not examined in any great detail.

The blood samples sent to Dr Owen had been put straight into the deep freeze without having first been separated into the clear fluid (serum) in which the red cells are suspended and the red cells themselves. This had caused the red cells to burst open, spilling the haemoglobin they contained into the serum and making it unsuitable for analysis for insulin or C-peptide. Dr Owen did try to analyse for insulin content the tissues that Dr Acland had removed surrounding the bruised area from the thigh, but found none. He concluded that while there was no obvious indication of an insulin overdose, he could not rule it out since he was unable to analyse the blood serum, owing to the way it had been treated.

The story does not end there, however. For reasons that are far from clear, a second set of post-mortem blood specimens was sent to the Newcastle specialist assay laboratory for analysis for insulin and C-peptide. So too were samples of urine from both the first and second post-mortems collected 5 days apart by Professor Jones and Dr Acland respectively. The blood samples, as Dr Owen had said, were not considered fit for analysis but the urine samples were, according to the advice of Dr Robin Ferner, the expert toxicologist the police had consulted in Birmingham.

The two urine samples, collected by Professor Jones and Dr Acland respectively, were given different identification codes when they were sent to the laboratory, and therefore were treated quite separately in the laboratory as though they were from different people.

They were reported to contain insulin at concentrations of 412 pmol/L and 197 pmol/L respectively: in other words, they were very different from one another even though they both came from the same deceased person's bladder, albeit 5 days apart. This raised the question of the reliability of the assay technique, and which measurement the court should use. The more than twofold difference in what was ostensibly the same sample did not arouse any concern in the laboratory that carried out the assay, and was unaware of it, nor in the prosecution – which was. It was only when the difference was pointed out to the prosecution by the defence shortly before the trial was scheduled to commence that it did. The corresponding concentrations of C-peptide in the two specimens were, as they might have been expected to be, roughly similar: 630 pmol/L and 580 pmol/L, respectively.

At that time, no one knew what the normal levels of insulin in urine from a dead body were. Not very much more was known about its concentration in urine collected during life from healthy people, because work undertaken by Dr Arthur Rubenstein, first in England but subsequently mainly in America, had suggested that it was too unreliable to have any clinical value. Dr Ferner, the expert advising the prosecution, very wisely, therefore, had arranged for urine to be collected anonymously from about 20 other corpses brought into mortuaries in Birmingham and analysed in the same laboratory in Newcastle and in the same batch as the two urine specimens from Eric.

Far more is known about the concentration of C-peptide in urine, as it has gained some popularity as a test for the integrity of the insulin-secreting pancreatic beta-cells in patients with type 1 diabetes, in whom some retention of function indicates a better prognosis than its complete loss. However, urinary C-peptide had never been measured in urine from a corpse. Results obtained for C-peptide on the urine samples from the control corpses collected in Birmingham and analysed in Newcastle were roughly similar to each other and to Eric's urine. However, the insulin concentration in Eric's urine was, depending on which result you believe, some 5–10 times higher than in the average of the control subjects.

The Newcastle laboratory had also received some of the blood samples collected from Eric post-mortem by Professor Jones and which, unknown to the analyst, represented two portions of the same sample put into two separate pots and given two different labels. The two samples were analysed for both C-peptide and insulin and were reported as containing 270 and 380 pmol/L of C-peptide and 35 and 16 pmol/L of insulin respectively. These are all perfectly normal but because the samples were haemolysed – that is coloured red because the red blood cells had broken down and released their haemoglobin into the serum – the insulin results were, quite rightly, discounted as they had been by Dr Owen in the forensic science laboratory. Scant attention was given to the C-peptide results, which, had they been accepted as valid – which they might reasonably have been since there is very little evidence on the stability of C-peptide in the presence of haemolysis – would virtually have eliminated the possibility that Eric's death was due to insulin-induced hypoglycaemia.

The West Midlands Police, the force investigating Eric's death, asked Dr Teale to comment on the results they had received from Newcastle. He expressed his concern about both the quality of the analytical procedures and their interpretation. The immunoassay kit that had been used to measure insulin had been designed and validated to measure insulin in blood plasma and serum, but not in urine. He pointed out that the results for insulin, but not for C-peptide, differed by more than 100% on what was, in effect, the same post-mortem sample. Dr Teale did not, himself, have any of the appropriate samples and therefore could not repeat the tests originally carried out in Newcastle on Eric's blood serum and urine and upon which so much depended. A minuscule amount of haemolysed serum was eventually found in the deep freeze some months later and an attempt was made to measure its C-peptide content, but none was found.

In his original contact with the West Midlands Police, Dr Teale had admitted that while he had extensive experience of the measurement of insulin, he would not claim to be an expert on the clinical interpretation of the results, especially those obtained only from urine. The main reason for his reticence was that the experts with the greatest experience of urinary insulin – and to a lesser extent C-peptide measurements – held that urinary insulin measurements are for various reasons uninterpretable and clinically worthless.

Dr Teale's opinion, which coincided with mine, did not accord, however, with that of Dr Robin Ferner, nor with the other people the police had consulted. By the time the case came to court the police had consulted a number of other experts and arranged for more urine samples to be collected from corpses under conditions more closely resembling those pertinent to Eric, such as similarity of time since death and age of the patient. The defence too had consulted experts, including me and Dr

Arthur Rubenstein of Chicago, who had also testified in the Claus von Bulow trial (see page 39).

The trial of Maria Whiston on a charge of murder by administration of insulin to Eric began in Birmingham Crown Court in the summer of 1996, more than 2 years after his death. It was then adjourned for more than 6 months and subsequently interrupted several times to permit further testing when the results of those that had already been carried out were challenged. Many more urine samples were collected from corpses and analysed in three of the country's leading immunoassay laboratories, Newcastle, Oxford and Guildford, but with only poor agreement as to their insulin and to a lesser extent their C-peptide content.

All the urine samples were, however, also measured for their creatinine content, in each of the three laboratories. Creatinine, a substance produced in the body at a more or less constant rate each day and excreted exclusively in urine, is measured routinely by a straightforward chemical reaction in all clinical laboratories for a number of reasons. The most common is as a test of kidney function; another is as a comparator or yardstick for other substances whose excretion is less predictable. The results for creatinine showed excellent agreement between the three laboratories – in contrast to their often marked disagreements with regard to urinary insulin and C-peptide measurements. This showed that the laboratories were performing properly but that the tests they used to measure insulin and C-peptide in urine were not particularly reliable. This cast serious doubt on the accuracy and reliability of these tests, upon which so much depended. Interpretation of the results was, of course, even more contentious, with prosecution and defence taking opposite viewpoints. The defence argued that the results could not be relied on for forensic purposes; the prosecution disagreed.

At trial the experts called by the two sides disagreed fundamentally on the significance of the urinary insulin and C-peptide results. They all gave scant attention to the insulin and C-peptide assays that had been performed on the blood, since both sides agreed that they were suspect.

Experts called by the defence included Dr Arthur Rubenstein, the undisputed world authority on urinary insulin measurements and their significance, Dr Derrick Teale, Head of the Immunoassay Department at the Royal Surrey County Hospital Guildford, Dr (now Professor) Linda Morgan, a distinguished endocrinologist and immunoassayist from the University of Surrey, and myself. We were all of the opinion that the results of the urinary insulin and C-peptide assays were uninterpretable even had they been accurate and agreed with one other. Experts consulted by the prosecution included Dr Robin Ferner, a distinguished forensic toxicologist and specialist in diabetes from Birmingham, the late

Professor Robert Turner of Oxford, one of the country's leading experts on diabetes and hypoglycaemia, and Professor Rury Holman, his successor in Oxford. They held a contrary opinion. They accepted not only that the analytical results for urinary insulin and C-peptide were accurate – or at least sufficiently so for the purpose – but also that they were consistent with, and indicative of, the administration of exogenous insulin from out of a bottle.

Professor Rubenstein, who felt so strongly about the case that he flew over from America for his day in court without fee, pointed out that the amounts of insulin and C-peptide excreted in the urine bear very little relationship to their concentration in the blood or to one another. This is because the kidneys handle them so very differently from one another and in different individuals. Even minor differences in kidney function can have a most profound effect on how much of the body's insulin finds its way into the urine. Ordinarily it is less than 0.1% but it can rise as high as 1–5%. Consequently neither the absolute concentration nor its concentration relative to that of C-peptide is any indication of the amount of insulin produced by or injected into the body each day.

Clinically it was impossible to rule out hypoglycaemia as the cause of Eric's death since, apart from certain changes that may occur in the microscopic anatomy of the brain, it cannot be diagnosed after death. The circumstances of his death were, however, odd, because vomiting, which was considered so important in the original investigation of his death, is almost unheard of in insulin-induced hypoglycaemia as both Dr Foster and I had testified in the Claus von Bulow case (see pages 26 and 42). Moreover, it usually takes a large amount of insulin and at least 24 hours to produce death predictably in an otherwise healthy person unless there is alcohol in the body, as in the Jane Wagstaffe case (see page 77), or there is something wrong with the patient's heart.

It emerged during her trial that on the night before finding Eric dead, Maria had not been on duty at the hospital, as she had said, but had spent the night with her current lover, Rodney Beattie. This was not the only lie that Maria had told. Maria had led Rodney to believe that she lived with a nursing friend, a Mrs Josebury, whose address and telephone number she gave as her own. Whilst Maria was on holiday in the Philippines during May 1994, Rodney, who had been Maria's lover since 1992, tried to contact her through the only address and telephone number he knew. It was only then that he learned of Maria's true relationship with Eric. She denied it and said the relationship was only a business one. Rodney clearly believed her and on her return from the Philippines they arranged to get married. Although he gave evidence for the prosecution, Rodney is quoted in a local newspaper as having said, of the charge against her,

"It's rubbish. She didn't do it. All the evidence is circumstantial. She is not capable of what they say she did".

A particularly telling witness for the prosecution was Maria's former husband, Robert Whiston, a company director from who she was divorced in 1990. He told the court that she had threatened, on one occasion, to kill him by injecting him with insulin between the toes where the marks would never be detected. This was presented as such a novel – and almost certainly incorrect – idea that the case became known in the media as the *"nurse who killed her lover by jabs between the toes"*. Dr Jaggit Sanghera, a former colleague of Maria's, said that she had joked to him about killing people with insulin and mentioned Beverly Allitt as an example. Constantine Terry, a prisoner who shared a cell with Maria while she was on remand, described how she admitted killing Eric and mentioned how people could also be killed by injecting them with air (see the Noburo Kato case, page 101).

Unbeknownst to anyone in the court except Robert, and possibly some of the lawyers, Maria had been heavily involved with the courts in the 2 years between Eric's death and her appearance in one as a defendant accused of his murder. This involvement had nothing to do with Eric but everything to do with Robert in a case that was to establish new principles in matrimonial law in England.

Robert had married Maria in England in June 1973. After 14 years, their relationship had deteriorated, and they separated in 1988. Robert was given custody of their two children a year later. Divorce proceedings were instituted but during these proceedings Robert learned that Maria was already married when she had married him.

Maria had married Vergilio Sabado in the Philippines in November 1962 and was still married to him when she went through a form of marriage with Robert. In January 1990 Robert was granted a decree of nullity on the grounds of Maria's bigamy.

What then followed was almost farcical. Maria had cross-applied in another court for something called ancillary relief. A judge sitting in the county court decided that Robert should pay her £25,000, which, on appeal, was reduced to £20,000. This is still a substantial amount and one that the Court of Appeal, the highest court in the country apart from the House of Lords, overturned when it considered the matter in March 1995. Their ruling established the law on this matter – probably forever more. The court's decision was based largely on the fact that no one should benefit from their own criminal activity, yet this is exactly what Maria's action in bigamously marrying Robert was. She had known full well that she was still married to Vergilio when she went through a wedding ceremony with Robert in 1973 even though she denied it under oath on at least two occasions during the custody and divorce proceedings before finally admitting it. This lying under oath, or perjury, did not go down well with the judges in the Court of Appeal, who did, however, do nothing further about it – possibly because they knew of the more serious charge against her that were shortly to be heard in the Crown Court in Birmingham.

Nothing of this was mentioned at Maria's trial for murder, of course, nor, somewhat surprisingly, did it feature in any of the often lurid descriptions of the case that appeared in the media in its aftermath.

Also produced in evidence at the trial was Eric's will. Had Eric's death gone unquestioned, Maria was the sole beneficiary and stood to inherit everything, including the house they jointly owned. It was Eric's daughter, Karen, who had been disinherited, who started the whole train of events that led to Maria's conviction. The sums involved were quite modest but the prosecution considered them sufficient a motive to be worth emphasizing in the case and in the closing statement. The jury appeared not to have been swayed by the argument that the scientific evidence that Eric's death was due to an insulin injection was seriously flawed. Though no injection sites were found despite a thorough search at post-mortem, and though the insulin analytical data were shaky, to say the least, this appeared to carry little weight with the jury, who convicted Maria of Eric's murder on Thursday 22nd May 1997.

Shortly after her conviction Maria sought leave to appeal. After first rejecting it, the court referred the case to the Criminal Cases Review Commission, who commissioned Professor David Owens, a very distinguished Professor of Diabetes Medicine in Cardiff, to review the case. He was clearly not very impressed by the scientific evidence implicating insulin in Eric's death and his report was referred to the Court of Appeal for further consideration.

The three judges constituting the Court of Appeal (Criminal Division) convened in London during July 2000 to consider the safety of Maria's conviction. The prosecution called a number of new experts, all of whom, like those at the original trial, believed that the scientific evidence implicated insulin in Eric's death. The defence called Dr Linda Morgan, from the University of Surrey, who confirmed what she had said at the original trial, and Dr Stuart Woodhead, an eminent immunoassayist with an international reputation, who said that the analyses for insulin performed on Eric's urine did not provide unequivocal evidence of insulin administration. In spite of this and Professor Owen's own reservations, the Court of Appeal ruled that the conviction was safe. The reason it gave was that all of the experts called by the defence, including me, volunteered the information that they could not categorically exclude the possibility that insulin had been administered even though they thought it unlikely. The results were therefore construed as consistent with the suggestion that insulin was responsible for Eric's death and the lower court's verdict upheld although the evidence for it, as Rodney Beattie said, was entirely circumstantial.

It is possible that Maria killed Eric, but I have doubts about the validity of the scientific evidence pointing to insulin as the weapon. Many other experts share these doubts – though not, apparently, the jury or the Court of Appeal. It is not hard to see why after reading their judgement. In it, the opinions expressed by Dr Rubenstein, undoubtedly the world's greatest authority on urinary insulin and C-peptide measurements, were considered no more valuable than those of witnesses with little or no previous experience of them. I was described as *"a slightly unusual and not particularly impressive witness"* and Dr Teale was not mentioned at all.

On 16th October 2002 an article appeared in *The Guardian* newspaper by an anonymous author who described the difficulties he had experienced in visiting Maria in Styal Prison. He said that he is so convinced of her innocence that he is preparing a website that will review her case and call for a retrial. It has not yet appeared.

9 Susan Shickle, England: "It wasn't me, it was him"

Norman Harvey was a frail 68-year-old man, living in rural Oxfordshire at the time of his death, sometime during the early morning of Friday 3rd May 1996. He was the legal tenant of a one-bedroom council flat, the use of which he shared in a complicated domestic arrangement with Susan Shickle, her lover and her daughter. Norman had known Susan Shickle, a 36-year-old divorcée, since she was a child, and had had a long, but intermittent and sexually ambiguous, relationship with her ever since. Susan, who had lived in the same block of flats but had recently been evicted, had moved into Norman's flat along with her lover, Mark Nash, and her young daughter.

Susan, having found Norman lying apparently dead on his bed, called the doctor to certify his death that spring morning. Later that day she was charged with his murder.

The police were already on site by the time the doctor arrived. Earlier that morning, Susan had telephoned her son Andrew to tell him she had killed Norman. Andrew told his father Stephen, Susan's former husband, and Stephen went to the police station with this information.

Dr George Mason, Norman's doctor, confirmed that he was dead but, after examining the body, said he had found nothing suspicious. Nevertheless, because Norman's death was sudden and unexpected, his body was taken to Horton General Hospital in Banbury, where a pathologist, Dr Joseph Sarvesvaran, carried out an autopsy at 3 pm that day.

Norman had been diagnosed as suffering from diabetes almost 20 years earlier, in January 1977, and initially put on oral medication with sulphonylurea tablets. This is a standard medicine for type 2 (previously known as late-onset) diabetes. He remained on the tablets until, in October 1992, his diabetes went out of control and he was put on twice-daily injections of insulin. Although he remained on twice-daily injections until January 1996, Norman appears to have been unusually susceptible to insulin's blood glucose-lowering properties. He had been admitted to

Horton General Hospital, in a hypoglycaemic coma on at least seven occasions during these 3½ years despite progressively reducing his dose of insulin and receiving supervision from the district nurse. On most of his admissions for hypoglycaemia from 1993 to 1995, Susan was recorded in his hospital case notes as his next of kin.

Norman's insulin treatment was discontinued on 24th January 1996 without apparent ill effect. This was done on the advice of Dr Peter Fisher, the hospital specialist, who had written to Norman's GP (Dr Mason) suggesting that, instead of insulin, he should use glibenclamide (an oral medication for diabetes) at a low dose of 2.5 mg a day, rising, if necessary, to 5 mg a day.

Norman's treatment with glibenclamide began on 8th February at a dose of 2.5 mg a day and was raised to 5 mg a day on his last visit to the clinic, on 22nd March 1996. Neither Dr Mason nor Dr Fisher prescribed him any insulin after January 1996. It was apparent to those looking after him that Norman was becoming increasingly frail. He had nevertheless kept an apparently accurate record of the insulin he gave himself right up to 24th January 1996, when, on doctor's advice, he stopped injecting it.

In his post-mortem report Dr Sarvesvaran described Norman as *"a frail elderly white male with recent puncture marks on the side of his left leg"*. They were situated about 130 cm below the level of his knee and surrounded by bruises from blood that had infiltrated the subcutaneous and muscular tissues. Dr Sarvesvaran removed the affected tissues together with some others that he considered might be injection sites so that they could be tested for insulin, along with blood samples.

Norman's body, Dr Sarvesvaran reported, had several other bruises. His heart was enlarged and his liver abnormal. His pancreas – the organ that makes insulin – was also abnormal. It was full of fibrous tissue and its duct contained stones, which was consistent with the history that Norman had previously suffered from an inflamed pancreas, and may have contributed to the onset of his diabetes. No detailed microscopic examination or immunoassay was made of any of the organs, and Norman's brain was not preserved for neuropathological examination.

Susan was arrested and charged with Norman's murder. At the request of the defence team, Dr Peter Jerreat, a Home Office Pathologist and Senior Forensic Medical Examiner to the City of London Police, carried out a second post-mortem on Norman's body on the afternoon of 14th May, 11 days after Norman died. Dr Jerreat also collected samples of tissue from the presumed insulin injection sites with a view to having them analysed for insulin using immunoassay. The body had been stored in a mortuary refrigerator, which would help preserve any insulin present in the tissues if it was there in the first place.

Dr Sarvesvaran had collected blood from a peripheral blood vessel at the first post-mortem and put it into a tube containing sodium fluoride. This is a standard preservative to prevent the destruction of glucose by the red cells in blood collected from a living person. It is not strictly necessary when blood is collected for analysis from a corpse since, for various reasons, post-mortem glucose measurements are virtually impossible to interpret anyway. The post-mortem sample of blood collected by Dr Sarvesvaran had a glucose concentration of 1.9 mmol/L, which, though low for a living person, is quite normal for someone who had been dead for more than a few hours. It provided no proof that Norman was suffering from hypoglycaemia at the time of his death.

Mr Allan Hiscutt, a Home Office Toxicologist, to whom all the samples collected at autopsy were originally sent, measured the glucose concentration of fluid taken from within the eyeball, the vitreous humour. This was unrecordably low, but again did not establish that Norman's blood glucose level had been low at the time of his death, though it would have eliminated the possibility of hypoglycaemia had it been normal or high. Serum from the blood collected from Norman's peripheral veins and arteries was also sent to the forensic science laboratory for insulin and C-peptide analysis. As Mr Hiscutt's laboratory did not have state-of-the-art facilities for measuring these two hormones, the samples were sent to the Guildford Supra-Regional Specialist Analytical Laboratory run by Dr Derrick Teale.

Dr Sarvesvaran had recorded the cause of death as insulin overdose, having heard the story elicited from two eyewitnesses: Andrew Shickle and one of his friends. He did not think the abnormalities he had found in Norman's heart and pancreas caused or contributed to Norman's death. Dr Jerreat, on the other hand, was less persuaded by the eyewitness accounts and believed that death might well have been due to natural causes. He cited as the probable cause the obviously severe lung and coronary heart disease that both he and Dr Sarvesvaran had observed at post-mortem.

When the case came to court in Oxford, Susan's 14-year-old son Andrew, who lived with her estranged husband, gave evidence. He and some of his school friends had been at Norman's house on the evening preceding his death. All gave similar stories. Two of the boys, including Andrew, had arrived at Norman's flat at about 6 pm and Susan let them in. They both noticed that she had been drinking cider – a pint glass of it had been very evident.

Fifteen or so minutes after the two boys arrived Norman returned home, took off his coat and went into his bedroom. He emerged again 30 minutes later. Susan asked him to go to the shop and buy a loaf of bread and a bottle of cider. She gave him some money but he did not go. This, the boy said, enraged Susan, who became increasingly angry, swearing and shouting at him as he continued to stay put. At this time two more of Andrew's friends arrived on the scene.

Shortly after their arrival, Susan, by this time seemingly extremely angry, threatened she would kill Norman if he came near her. Norman retired to the bedroom once again. Sometime during the next half hour or so, Susan picked up some syringes she had available and drew up liquid from a vial that the witnesses said was insulin.

Susan then went into Norman's bedroom where she stayed for a few minutes. During the next hour or so Norman came out of his bedroom once or twice, but on each occasion Susan pushed him back into it. Immediately preceding each occasion she was said to have filled another syringe with insulin from a vial and followed him into the bedroom. The last time Norman came out of his room, Susan was seen to inject him in the leg with the fluid from the syringe she was holding.

After Norman had returned to his room for the last time, Susan instructed her son to fetch her lover, Mark Nash, from a friend's house where he was spending the evening. Nash returned to the flat, but found Susan in such a foul mood that he quickly left and did not return to sleep there until about 4 am. Next morning he woke up to hear Susan saying that she had found Norman dead in his bed.

Mr Hiscutt examined the various specimens collected at autopsy but found no alcohol in any of them. He did, however, find significant amounts of three types of benzodiazepines – drugs used as tranquillizers or sleeping pills. None was present in lethal amount and while he thought it technically possible that only one of them, diazepam, had actually been swallowed – as the other two are both capable of being produced from it by metabolism in the body – he thought it more likely that Norman had taken, or been given, both diazepam and temazepam some hours before his death.

In addition to routine analysis of the serum samples from post-mortem blood for drugs, Mr Hiscutt, as he had been asked, also measured the insulin content using a commercial radioimmunoassay kit in his laboratory. The sample contained 6090 pmol/L (812 µU/ml). This is a very high figure – anything over 2000 pmol/L is suspicious of insulin misuse – and because he was not himself an expert in insulin analysis he had, on 15th May 1996, sent some of the sample on to Dr Teale. He also sent him some of the tissues Dr Sarvesvaran and Dr Jerreat had removed from Norman's body at post-mortem and which they believed might have been the injection sites.

The clinical laboratory in Guildford where Dr Teale worked as the biochemist in charge has an international reputation for the investigation of hypoglycaemia. It is a reference centre for much of the UK, receiving samples for analysis from around the country. It was one of the pioneer laboratories in the application of insulin, C-peptide and pro-insulin (the substance in the body from which insulin is made) immunoassays to clinical problems associated with hypoglycaemia.

Dr Teale used a radioimmunoassay system based on the original technique developed by Yalow and Berson to measure insulin in the samples he received (see page 14). It was similar to the one employed by Mr Hiscutt but with slight variations – it used a different antiserum and a slightly different protocol, for example. Dr Teale also used a more sophisticated technique known as serial dilution (previously described on page 69) in which increasingly small amounts of the sample are analysed, since when concentrations are very high in the original sample this is the only way to produce an accurate result.

In Guildford the serum sample collected from Norman was found to contain insulin at a concentration of 11,500 pmol/L, or some 100–500 times the level usually found in someone who has not eaten recently. It was almost twice as high as Mr Hiscutt had found using the less sophisticated technique.

Dr Teale's attempts to measure C-peptide in the sample were unsuccessful as there was insufficient C-peptide present to detect by the radioimmunoassay – as there undoubtedly would have been if the insulin he had found in the serum sample had come from Norman's own pancreas instead of from a syringe. Taken together these two observations – high insulin but absent C-peptide – are highly suggestive, though not absolutely diagnostic, of hypoglycaemia resulting from the administration of pharmaceutical insulin.

Dr Teale analysed for their insulin content the tissue removed from Norman's body at each of the two autopsies. He received no tissues from parts of the body that were believed not to have been injected and which would have been useful for comparison with sites that were.

None of the samples of tissues removed at the second autopsy by Dr Jerreat contained any insulin. This may have been due to a failure to sample an actual injection site or simply due to the destruction of insulin in the body, and of course the blood it contained, with the passage of time.

Nevertheless the tissues removed at the first autopsy (performed by Dr Sarvesvaran) did contain insulin at a comparatively low concentration of 309 pmol/kg in the sample from one injection site and of 67 pmol/kg in that from the other. These results are difficult to interpret as they may have been contaminated by blood, which was already known to have very high insulin levels.

Mr Hiscutt's and Dr Teale's results on the post-mortem serum samples and the conclusions based upon them were regarded as crucial by the experts called by the prosecution, of which I was one, and were presented by them to the court as supporting evidence of malicious insulin administration.

The defence called Dr Patrick Toseland, a Consultant Clinical Biochemist and Toxicologist from Guy's Hospital Medical School in London with extensive experience of insulin poisoning, to contradict our evidence. He pointed to the marked discrepancy in the values for serum insulin obtained on the same sample by Mr Hiscutt and Dr Teale and wondered which of them, if either, was correct. He also drew attention to the fact that neither analyst had specifically excluded the possibility of interference from insulin antibodies, which might have been present in Norman's blood from his previous legitimate use of insulin. Dr Toseland, also quite rightly, did not accept Dr Teale's contention that serial dilution absolutely excluded the possibility of interference in the insulin assay (see Deborah Winzar case, page 127), the results of which might therefore have been totally incorrect.

Dr Toseland questioned the significance of the modest insulin levels found in extracts of the tissues removed from the purported injection sites. They were not compared with the insulin content of tissues far removed from possible injection sites, and the concentrations found were many times lower than those reported by analysts in the Kenneth Barlow case (see page 4) and other well-documented murder cases in which an insulin injection site had been identified.

During enquires made by the police prior to charging Susan with murder on 24th May 1996, it emerged that a certain Jeffrey Ball had been convicted earlier that year at Oxford Crown Court on a charge of causing her actual bodily harm. He apparently told his solicitor in February 1996 that he had, on a previous occasion, seen her maliciously inject Norman with insulin. The prosecution declined to call him as a witness, however, as he had been such a poor witness at his own trial that the value of his evidence was suspect.

A curious twist to the case occurred when the defence team claimed that it was not Susan but her son, Andrew, who had injected the insulin that killed Norman. The jury did not believe this and on 25th February 1997 Susan was found guilty at Oxford Crown Court of murdering Norman and sentenced to life imprisonment. Her appeal against the conviction was dismissed in July 1997. More recently the Criminal Cases Review Commission, to whom it was referred in May 2001, recommended a referral to the Court of Appeal, having itself considered new evidence relating to her psychological state at the time of the offence. The appeal was heard at The Royal Courts of Justice in London and dismissed on 14th July 2005.

10 Noburo Kato*, Japan: a botched murder

Noburo Kato was 25 when he died at home in the winter of 1999 surrounded by several vials of insulin and some tranquillizer tablets.

The police were notified of his unexpected death and took his body to the Forensic Medicine Department of the Graduate School of Medicine of Tokyo University for investigation into the cause of his death. On the evidence before them, they suspected, not unreasonably, that this was caused by an insulin overdose that he had probably administered himself.

At the post-mortem examination, carried out some 30 hours after his death, the pathologist found that air rather than blood filled the right side of the heart and that the small blood vessels of the lungs were blocked by air bubbles. It was clear that at least 50 ml of air had been injected into his veins and that this, and not insulin, was the immediate cause of his death. It also virtually ruled out suicide, as it would be extremely difficult for an individual to inject himself with that amount of air intravenously.

Noburo's girl friend (I do not know whether he was married), who was a nurse, was the obvious main suspect, and when confronted with the evidence she confessed to murdering him and described how she went about it. She began by giving Noburo a drink of fruit juice containing triazolam, a tranquillizer. She proceeded to set up an intravenous drip containing glucose in his left arm, into which she then administered 30 mg of diazepam (Valium), 20 mg of reserpine (an old-fashioned drug used to lower the blood pressure) and 1200 units of long-acting insulin. This cocktail of drugs did not, however, kill him quickly enough for her purposes so she then injected him with about 100 ml of air, which did.

Her account of the insulin injection was substantiated by the finding of a disproportionately high plasma insulin-to-C-peptide ratio in the blood collected from the right side of Noburo's heart. Neither the concentration of insulin (388 pmol/L) nor that of C-peptide (166 pmol/

---

* Not his real name.

L) was diagnostically high and would not have been considered remarkable under different circumstances, especially as the blood was collected from the right side of the heart and might have been contaminated by insulin and C-peptide diffusing into it from the pancreas. The C-peptide-to-insulin ratio was, however, only 0.5:1 (i.e. twice as much insulin as C-peptide), compared with a more usual figure of about 6:1 (i.e. six times as much C-peptide as insulin) in living people and 20:1 in corpses, and consistent with a story of insulin poisoning. If the results of the insulin and C-peptide assays had been the only evidence, they would probably not have been sufficient to substantiate a charge of malicious insulin administration. However, those results, together with the circumstantial evidence provided by the empty insulin vials, the defendant's confession and the post-mortem findings of air in Noburo's heart and lungs, were sufficient to secure his lover's conviction of murder, for which she received a long custodial sentence. No motive or explanation emerged for the amazingly elaborate steps she took to kill Noburo. These are reminiscent of the steps taken by Herr Breslau and his mistress to kill his wife some 50 years ago (see page 8).

What is remarkable about this case is how rapidly the huge dose of insulin given intravenously disappeared from the circulation after it had been injected. Had the same amount been given into the tissues, as is usually the case, it would undoubtedly have been present in post-mortem blood at a concentration of thousands if not tens of thousands, of picomoles per litre.

11 Deborah Winzar, England: a case of wrongful conviction?

Deborah Winzar, known to all her friends as Dee, had been married to Dominic McCarthy (usually known as Nic) for 12 years when she stood trial in Birmingham in the summer of 2000 accused of his murder.

Nic was 34 years old, Dee was 2 years younger. They had met when they were trainee nurses and established a stable relationship early in 1984. On 25th October 1984 Nic was involved in a motorbike accident that left him paraplegic, but he and Dee went ahead as planned and were married on 19th January 1985.

Nic was awarded £675,000 compensation in 1991 for the injuries that he suffered, and the couple moved to Cambridgeshire. Dee became a nursing sister at a hospital 20 miles away from their home and Nic continued working as a social worker. So far as can be ascertained, they lived a happy conjugal life, which resulted in the birth of their son, Tony, in 1995.

On 31st January 1997 Nic was found unconscious on his bed at home whilst Dee was at work. He died 9 days later.

I was approached, some 19 month later, on 1st September 1998, by Dee's then solicitor, Philip Eldin-Taylor, and asked to review the papers and offer an expert opinion on them.

Dee had recently been charged with murdering Nic by injecting him with insulin at an unspecified time on either the evening of 30th January or the morning of 31st January 1997. The case was first heard at Peterborough Magistrates Court on 5th August 1998 and referred to the Crown Court at Northampton for trial, but it was not until July 2000, no less than 3½ years after the event, that Dee was convicted of Nic's murder in Birmingham Crown Court.

I accepted Philip Eldin-Taylor's request but declared an interest. I already knew something about the case because Dr Derrick Teale, Chief Biochemist in my old laboratory in Guildford, which was a National

Reference Centre for insulin measurement and to which I still acted as a consultant, had carried out the crucial insulin and C-peptide assays. The whole case depended on the accuracy of these tests and I might therefore be biased in their favour. I also said, in my preliminary communication, that my impression was that either Nic himself, or another person, had given insulin in an amount sufficient to produce hypoglycaemia but that I had nothing more to go on than the laboratory results. I had no clinical notes. I added that, contrary to popular belief, the interpretation of laboratory data is never self-evident and must be made against a full examination of the circumstances. This is because laboratory results can sometimes, though rarely, be misleading by giving falsely positive and falsely negative results. In the clinic this can lead to an incorrect diagnosis, and in a court of law to people who are innocent being found guilty and those who are guilty as innocent.

I said that although I would accept the brief, I could not be very encouraging since, on the face of it, the results pointed to administration of insulin as the cause of the hypoglycaemia. I did, however, point out that self-administration of insulin with suicidal intent was many times more common than murder with it – but until I had had a chance to look at all the evidence I could say no more. All I knew, at that time, was that Nic had been admitted to hospital suffering from hypoglycaemic coma on 31st January 1997 and that the ratio of insulin to C-peptide found in the samples taken from him suggested that the insulin in his blood had come from a source other than his own pancreas. Later, after reviewing the evidence, I realized that my original opinion, based on inadequate information, was wrong. Nic had almost certainly never been injected with insulin, though, as so often happens in medicine, it was impossible to disprove the possibility that he had.

I received the papers – all 4 kg of them. They consisted of all of Nic's clinical notes and witness statements from 23 people, including an expert, Dr (now Professor) Robert Forrest, who had been consulted by the prosecution. He had seen all the data upon which the case against Dee was based; I had not. Dr Forrest knew that as an expert witness his duty was to help the court and not to advocate a cause or favour his client, who, in this case, was the police. His impartial report, written on 14th April 1997, just 3 months after Nic's death, concluded that Nic's hypoglycaemia was caused by insulin – though it was not his responsibility to say who might have administered it. It was he who advised the defence to consult me. His report was helpful to me in highlighting some of the issues that I needed to address.

Soon after launching into my reading of Nic's clinical case notes I changed my mind from thinking that his hypoglycaemia – about which there was no doubt – was caused by insulin, to being pretty sure that it was not. I could not be certain – you so rarely can be in the practice of clinical medicine. I found myself increasingly inclined to support the view expressed in the clinical notes made at 10 pm on the day of his death, 9th February 1997, by Assistant Nurse Amphlett that, *"We still do not know what caused Nic's hypoglycaemia, Matsiko* [the consultant physician] *suspects septicaemia but Anthony* [Dr Brooks, a consultant anaesthetist] *is doubtful"*. I was impressed that Dr Katono Matsiko, a general physician, was aware that septicaemia could cause hypoglycaemia, as it was thought to do so only in patients with liver disease. It is only more recently that it has been shown that severe infection can cause hypoglycaemia in anyone, whether or not they have liver disease.

The record, made before the insulin assay results were to hand, was made in a section of the notes called "communication with relatives". It was dated and timed 10 hours after Nic had died and purported to be the record of an earlier meeting between Dr Books, Dee and one of Nic's sisters in law. They were told that his *"chest condition seems to be getting worse"* and *"his prognosis remains poor* [sic] *but it is probable that the only organ he will be able to donate are his corneas"*. The note concluded with the statement *"Blood cultures were not obtained on admission. Initial results do not point to an insulin overdose but we are still waiting for results from Guildford. These should arrive next week. The need for a possible coroner's case was discussed"*.

Although paraplegic, Nic was mobile in a wheelchair and was considered by his GP and by himself as *"medically fit"*. He was holding down a responsible job as a social worker and drove a suitably adapted car with no difficulty. Physically he was very powerful above the waist – but paralysed below it with absolutely no sensation or sense of touch. He was a bodybuilding enthusiast and regularly undertook weight training, but he was grossly overweight. He weighed 127 kg (20 stone), was 1.83 m (6 ft 1 in) tall and had a body mass index (BMI) of 38. The normal range is 18–25. A BMI of over 25 is defined as overweight and one of more than 30 as obese.

Nic's injury to his spinal cord had destroyed his bladder control and he had an indwelling catheter inserted into his bladder through his penis that enabled him to collect urine in a bag strapped unobtrusively to his thigh and which he could empty from time to time. The catheter, named after its inventor, a Dr Foley, was prevented from slipping out of the bladder by a little balloon that surrounded its tip. This was inflated with saline through a syringe when the catheter was inserted, and deflated when it was removed. Both Nic and his wife were able to do this. Unfortunately, indwelling catheters are not good at keeping germs out of

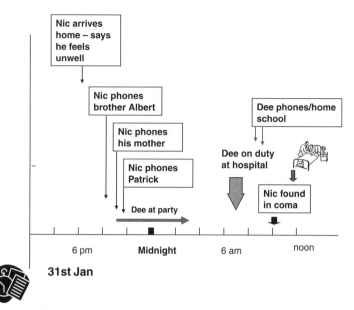

Figure 14 Sequence of events leading up to Nic McCarthy being found in a coma.

the bladder, and Nic suffered from intermittent bladder infections, for which he needed antibiotics.

The events that led to Dee's indictment for murder began on the evening of 30th January 1997 when she left the marital home to go to a party run by the junior doctors at the hospital where she worked, calling on the way to pick up a nursing friend, Mary Newell. Nic stayed at home to look after their son Tony as he had done many times before. Nic had said he was not feeling too well but that he would be all right and that Dee should go to the party as agreed.

It was arranged that Dee would stay with Mary Newell overnight as she was on duty at 7 am next morning. Mary lived near the hospital, which was about 45 minutes drive from Dee's house. Dee phoned Mary from her car around 8.50 pm to say she was on her way, and arrived at Mary's house about 9.10 pm. She must therefore have left the house no later than 8.45 pm.

Shortly before Dee left home that evening Nic had a telephone conversation with his older brother, Albert, around 8.15 pm and said he felt very tired. He spoke to his mother, also by phone, at around 9.06 pm, shortly after Dee left, but did not mention the tiredness. At around 9.10

pm Nic phoned another brother, Patrick, and spoke to him for about 10 minutes, ending by saying that he felt very tired and was going to bed.

The next morning, at about 9.50 am, Jane Lancaster-Adlam, Tony's kindergarten teacher, discovered Nic lying naked and unconscious on his bed. Because at Dee's trial a couple of years later great importance was attached to the events leading up to this discovery, it is necessary to describe them in some detail.

Jane offered to go to the McCarthy house because Tony had failed to materialize at the nursery school and Dee was clearly concerned because she had received no reply from Nic when she had tried to phone him at work, then on his car phone and finally at home. Ordinarily Tony was delivered to the nursery by one of his parents at around 8.30 am.

On this morning, presumably because Nic had been poorly before she left for the party and she had been unable to raise him on his own phone, Dee had phoned the school around 9.00 am to find out if he had arrived. She was told that he had not. Dee phoned again at about 9.20 am and this time spoke to Jane herself. Dee said she had tried to get Nic on the house and car phones but without success. Jane offered to go round to their house to see if there was a problem.

When she arrived at the McCarthy's home, Jane noticed Nic's Mercedes in the drive and assumed that he had overslept. Her initial knocking and increasingly desperate hammering on the door went unanswered. Putting her hand through the letterbox, she saw Tony standing next to the door. She spoke to him and asked him where his daddy was. Tony replied that daddy was upstairs sleeping and that he could not wake him up. Jane asked him to try again but he returned to say he still couldn't wake his daddy up. Jane then persuaded Tony to pass the house keys to her through the letterbox and she entered the house. She asked Tony to show her where his daddy was. On entering his bedroom upstairs Jane saw Nic lying naked and apparently asleep facing away from her. Overcoming her embarrassment, she tried to wake him without success. She then phoned Dee at work to tell her what she had found; Dee had left her phone number when they had spoken a few minutes earlier. At Dee's suggestion, Jane phoned their GP, Dr Roberts, who knew them all very well and whose surgery was just round the corner in the next village. Jane got straight through to Dr Roberts, who dropped what he was doing and came round to the McCarthy's house immediately.

Dr Roberts later said in his witness statement that he found Nic lying naked on his back on the bed. He described Nic's skin as *"slightly cold to touch though the room was warm"* and his breathing as laboured. He said Nic's lungs *"sounded bubbly"*. Dr Robert's first impression was that

Nic might have inhaled vomit and rang for an ambulance for his immediate transfer to hospital. He did not actually see any evidence of vomiting at that stage, although later, when eventually Nic was moved by the ambulance crew, he did vomit.

The ambulance crew arrived within minutes of being called and one of them asked Dr Roberts to put a plastic venous access line (a Venflon) into one of Nic's veins. This he did, but with difficulty and with some blood escaping, staining what he described as a previously un-bloodstained sheet. Dee arrived before Dr Roberts left (at 10.40 am) and whilst the ambulance crew were attending to her husband.

Dr Roberts observed that, *"Nic's catheter bag was bursting full"* when he arrived on the scene and that *"Debora emptied the bag as opposed to changing it"* soon after she arrived. The ambulance officer, Julie Hill, confirmed this. Much was made of Dee's action at the trial as if she was trying to conceal something, yet it was a natural and sensible thing to do. The implication was that Dee had attempted to dispose of evidence of poisoning by getting rid of Nic's urine.

Dr Roberts noticed a small (orange) 25-gauge needle lying opposite the bedroom door. This needle was subsequently tested for insulin after Dee had been charged with Nic's murder, but none was found on it. Because of the discovery of the needle, Dr Roberts had *"a cursory look round the bedroom"* but could not see any syringes or anything that he felt relevant to Nic's condition. Nor could the ambulance crew, who also *"looked around the room for a syringe but couldn't find one"*.

At the time when he became ill with hypoglycaemia Nic was receiving treatment with baclofen, a drug used to prevent muscle spasm from which he was suffering whenever his lower limbs were touched; Ditropan (oxybutynin), a drug that helps to prevent bladder spasms; and Gaviscon, an indigestion medicine. None was given by injection.

The ambulance crew continued, while taking him to hospital, to give Nic the oxygen commenced by Dr Roberts. Whether this was because he was blue from lack of oxygen or because they did it routinely is unclear. This distinction is important because severe and prolonged oxygen shortage can itself cause hypoglycaemia by interfering with the liver's ability to make glucose.

Because of Nic's weight, the first crew summoned a second crew to help take him downstairs on a stretcher and get him into an ambulance. When they got him into the ambulance Mr McSorley, one of the crew, had attempted to sit Nic upright. He vomited, but whether for the first time or for the second time, as Dr Roberts' statements imply, is unclear. Mr McSorley said he did not recollect seeing any vomit on the undersheet or on the quilt when he arrived. Dr Robert's had stated quite categorically that the sheets were not bloodstained when he arrived but when asked about it later could not recall if vomit was present. Nevertheless he acted on the supposition that Nic had vomited and that his immediate distress was due to its inhalation.

The ambulance crew attempted to measure Nic's blood pressure whilst he was on his way to the hospital. The systolic blood pressure (the higher of the two measurements of blood pressure) was recorded as being 110 mmHg, which is normal, but the diastolic blood pressure, the lower – and in many respects the more important of the two measurements – was not recorded. Whether this was because it was so low as to be unrecordable, or because it just was not measured, is unclear. The first blood pressure measurement made on his arrival in hospital at 12.30 pm appears to have been 132/64 mmHg. This was pretty much his normal blood pressure, and not very different from his last recorded blood pressure measurement of 130/80 mmHg made by his GP. The only other relevant information contained in Nic's GP notes was his susceptibility to recurrent bladder infections, for which he required antibiotics. This is commonplace in people with indwelling catheters.

Whilst in the ambulance Nic was given an intravenous injection of diazepam, a powerful tranquillizer, because he was thought to have been suffering from a fit – although he might merely have been having one of his muscular spasms, for which he was receiving treatment from his doctor. Mr Allan Hiscutt, a Home Office Toxicologist, subsequently detected diazepam, but no other benzodiazepine tranquillizers, in Nic's urine.

On arrival at the A&E Department* of Hinchinbrooke Hospital in Huntingdon, Nic was deeply comatose; he was grade 3 on the Glasgow Coma Scale, which ranges from 3 to 15, or, to put it another way, as profoundly unconscious as it is possible to be and still be alive. Earlier Dr Roberts had described him as capable of responding to pain, which in my experience is unheard of in someone in irreversible hypoglycaemic coma.

Mr Ernest Okagbue, a surgeon who was the A&E doctor on duty, said Nic had *"remnants of vomit on his clothing"*, but what bits of clothing was never specified; it will be recalled that he was described as naked when Jane, and subsequently Dr Roberts, found him.

Nothing pointed to Nic suffering from hypoglycaemia until a routine blood glucose test undertaken in the A&E Department revealed it. As soon as he saw the result, Mr Okagbue put another cannula into one of Nic's veins and collected blood for later analysis in the laboratory. He

---

* Emergency Room in America.

then injected 50 ml of 50% glucose (25 g) followed soon after by another injection of the same size. Neither injection had any significant effect upon Nic's level of consciousness – which they probably would have done if Nic was able to respond to a painful stimulus as Dr Roberts described, and had been in hypoglycaemic coma for less than 8 hours as the Court of Appeal was, much later, to find.

Mr Okagbue made it very clear that he and Dee, who arrived at the hospital in the ambulance with Nic, did not see eye to eye about the quality of care he was receiving in the A&E Department even though this was the first time they had met. Dee apparently expressed the view that a specialist physician rather than a surgeon should be looking after Nic. This might be thought not to be the behaviour of someone who wanted her husband to die, but, perhaps not surprisingly, was not well received by Mr Okagbue, who nevertheless subsequently acquiesced. He later made his feelings clear by telling the police that Dee *"did not seem to have the normal compassionate manner of a grieving relative"*.

By the time of his first glucose injection at about midday, Nic had been in a coma for more than 3 hours but almost certainly less than 8 hours. Failure to recover from hypoglycaemic coma of this duration after starting adequate glucose therapy is unusual and should lead to consideration of other causes of coma. It may have been Mr Okagbue's lack of curiosity as to the cause of her husband's unexpected illness, and its obvious seriousness, that led Dee to suggest that a specialist physician should see her husband. In Nic's case Dr Matsiko appears to have thought, at least initially, that Nic's hypoglycaemia was possibly a consequence, rather than the cause, of his illness.

In the period between Nic's admission to hospital and his death 9 days later he received appropriate supportive therapy. For the first 24 hours this involved treatment with intravenous glucose in amounts sufficient to keep his blood glucose within the normal range. According to the hospital's clinical notes, he received three glucose injections during his first 24 hours in hospital. Each was of 25 g, and he received a further 25–50 g of glucose through a continuous intravenous drip. In all he probably received about 150 g of glucose during his first day in hospital, but it might have been as high as 250 g; it was almost certainly not more than this. Had he received a fatal dose of insulin, he would probably have needed more glucose than this to bring his blood sugar up to normal and keep it there.

The assumption that Nic had inhaled vomit was a reasonable one based on the clinical history and the presence of vomit on his person and around his mouth. Because of this tentative diagnosis by Dr Roberts, Nic was, very soon after his arrival at Hinchinbrooke Hospital, put on a course of treatment with powerful antibiotics in addition to general supportive therapy and the intravenous glucose. The effect of this treatment, especially the antibiotics, would, however, have obscured any subsequent laboratory evidence of a serious infection. This might have arisen from his indwelling catheter or some unrelated virulent infection, such as meningitis, and been responsible for his illness. It would also explain why, on the night Dee went to the party, Nic had told his family he felt tired and went to bed early. Since, as the Court of Appeal found, the "insulin injection" could not have been given before the party, the "tiredness" that Nic had reported to his family that evening must have had some other, unrelated, cause and was not the early effect of an injection of insulin.

A blood culture was undertaken to determine whether Nic might have been suffering from septicaemia – but not until after he had already started on antibiotic therapy. Not surprisingly, the blood culture showed nothing – because the antibiotics he had already been given would have killed off the bacteria responsible if they had been there.

Nic's condition continued to deteriorate during the whole of the 9 days he survived. During much of this time, he was treated as someone with possible irreversible and ultimately fatal brain damage due to swelling of the brain – identified by a CAT scan made within an hour of his arrival at Hinchinbrooke Hospital. Eventually he was pronounced brain-dead and the life support machinery was switched off. Frequent meetings were held by the clinical staff with Dee and with Nic's family throughout his hospital stay. All were adamant that Nic would not have attempted to take his own life. Dee had also told the ambulance crew this on the day of the onset of Nic's illness. As with the concern expressed by Dee about the appropriateness of the care that Mr Okagbue was able to provide for Nic, this might seem to be somewhat inconsistent with the behaviour that might have been expected had Dee indeed tried to harm him.

Dr Roberts' contemporaneous notes – made long before there was any suspicion of foul play – describe Nic, when he was first discovered, as having "*bubbling chest and grey: seriously ill: given oxygen, ambulance called, aspirated and* [I] *inserted a Venflon*". This means that he sucked out vomit/fluid from Nic's windpipe and put a plastic cannula into a vein to facilitate collecting blood or injecting intravenous fluids. Inhalation of vomit due to hypoglycaemia was the working diagnosis right up to the time of Nic's death, though other possibilities were not ruled out.

Blood was collected from Nic immediately on his arrival in A&E and before the injection of glucose. It arrived in the laboratory at about midday with a request for analysis for glucose, urea and electrolytes, liver function tests, and cardiac enzymes. There was no request for analyses for insulin and C-peptide at that time, but later in the afternoon, at 2.50 pm to be precise, Dr Matsiko – the physician who had by this time taken over responsibility for Nic's treatment – did make a request. He also asked the laboratory to look for sulphonylureas in urine. These are medicines used to treat diabetes that can cause hypoglycaemia when taken by mouth and can easily be detected both in blood and urine when taken even in therapeutic amounts.

Hypoglycaemia caused by insulin or sulphonylurea remained high on the list of possible diagnoses as late as 9th February, the day Nic died. Dr Matsiko apparently still held to the view, according to the contemporaneous clinical notes, that the illness might have been due to septicaemia. Another possibility was insulinoma – an insulin-secreting tumour of the pancreas – but this was now deemed unlikely because of the lack of any further hypoglycaemic episodes; that is, once Nic's blood glucose level was restored to normal, it stayed there.

It seems likely, but was nowhere specifically stated or confirmed, that the sample of blood analysed for its insulin and C-peptide content in the Supra Regional Assay (Reference) Laboratory in Guildford was the one collected before Nic was given any intravenous glucose.

The Guildford laboratory, run by Dr Derrick Teale, always measured the glucose level in samples analysed for insulin and C-peptide content to ensure that the patient really was hypoglycaemic at the time the blood was collected. Without this simultaneous measurement, interpretation of insulin and C-peptide results can be extremely difficult. The glucose concentration in the sample of Nic's blood that Dr Teale analysed was 0.7 mmol/L. This is very low, but its cause could only be determined by measuring the insulin and C-peptide concentrations in the sample – and then only with caution. If the hypoglycaemia was due to an insulin injection, not only would the plasma insulin level be high but the C-peptide level would be low: if it was due to an insulin-secreting tumour or sulphonylurea ingestion, both would be high. With most other causes of hypoglycaemia, both insulin and C-peptide would be low.

In the event, the results of analysis on the blood sample showed an inappropriately high plasma insulin and a low plasma C-peptide level; this is the only hard, if not sole, piece of evidence upon which Dee's conviction for murder depends. The urine sample did not contain any sulphonylureas, thereby ruling out the possibility that Nic had taken any of these drugs.

The urine did, however, contain both insulin and C-peptide. These would not ordinarily have been measured – because they are virtually uninterpretable (as is described in the Maria Whiston case, page 89). They were, however, measured out of curiosity on this occasion because, in the absence of any clinical data, both Dr Teale and I assumed this to be a case of insulin-induced hypoglycaemia and were, by coincidence, both involved in the Maria Whiston case whose trial was proceeding at the very time that Nic's specimens arrived in Guildford. The results were, as we both knew they would be, uninterpretable, but they might possibly be useful for future reference in other cases of unexplained hypoglycaemia. The tests were undertaken long before there was any question of criminal proceedings. In Nic's case the presence of substantial amounts of C-peptide in his urine suggests that the insulin that accompanied it was from his own pancreas rather than exogenous. It is no more than a suggestion, as there is no experimental evidence on this point. It turned out, however, that the sample sent for analysis might have been collected after rather than before Nic had been given glucose. No one could be sure, and so the results were worthless.

The assays requested on Nic's blood were not considered urgent and it took 10 days for the results to be returned to the clinical staff at Hinchinbrooke Hospital. However, I doubt that Nic would have received any different treatment – or that a different clinical outcome would have been achieved – had the results become available immediately.

When they became available, Dr Teale very properly reported his results as *"consistent"* with exogenous insulin administration – which they are – and probably added the rider, as I would myself in the absence of any clinical information, that they were highly suggestive of it. I should perhaps explain here that, in my experience, laboratory doctors use the term "consistent with" differently from lawyers. Doctors imply by "consistent with" that the results do not rule out a possible diagnosis if it seems likely on other evidence; lawyers appear to use it to mean that the diagnosis is likely or "ruled in".

As was routine in the laboratory, Dr Teale kept the remaining plasma in the deep freeze in case other tests might be required. Because the results suggested that Nic's hypoglycaemia was due to insulin administration, the police were informed. They arranged for the deep frozen plasma sample to be taken to Mr Hiscutt, a Home Office Toxicologist, for further analysis.

In addition to a number of toxicological examinations, Mr Hiscutt analysed the plasma sample for insulin and C-peptide, though he acknowledged that, unlike Dr Teale, this was not his special area of expertise. The results he obtained, though similar to Dr Teale's for C-peptide (87 versus less than 94 pmol/L, the lowest limit of detection), were sufficiently different in the case of insulin (616 versus 887 pmol/L, i.e. some 30%) to throw doubt on the validity of both sets of results.

Very few other tests were done on Nic during the rest of his hospital admission that could have thrown light on the cause of his hypoglycaemia. There was, however, one thing that struck me as important – though it received scant attention while he was alive and was not taken seriously by the medical experts called by the prosecution to give evidence at Dee's trial. It was that, as part of their routine care, the doctors looking after Nic requested a range of routine biochemical tests every day. These included tests of liver function. Only one of these was glaringly abnormal – and then only when looked at over the course of time. It was his plasma albumin concentration. This had been perfectly normal at 39 g/L on the day he was admitted to hospital, but had fallen by a third to 29 g/L after only 24 hours, and to half, i.e. 20 g/L, on day 4 of his hospital stay. Such a rapid drop can only occur through loss of albumin from the blood into the tissues by increased leakage through the tiny blood vessels known as capillaries. It characteristically occurs only in very severe infections or surgical shock; it does not, as far as I can ascertain, occur in straightforward insulin-induced coma.

During Dee's trial, I gave, as my expert opinion, the view that Nic was the victim of a spontaneous and very profound illness and that his hypoglycaemia was part of this and not its cause. None of the experts called by the prosecution who addressed the possibility that his primary illness might have been a severe infection was asked to discuss the rapid drop in his plasma albumin levels and its causes. Since Dee's trial, I have had the opportunity of discussing it with one of the world's experts on the interpretation of plasma albumin assays, and he is firmly of the opinion that the only cause for such a rapid fall in plasma albumin concentration is its loss into the tissues by leakage through the capillaries.

Dr Michael Harris, the hospital pathologist, carried out a post-mortem examination on Nic's body on 11th February. He had already learned of Dr Teale's insulin assay results. The autopsy established that Nic's death was due to adult respiratory distress syndrome. That was as far as his own findings permitted him to go, but in the light of the clinical history he concluded that it was probably due to inhalation of vomit. This, in turn, based on Dr Teale's results, he attributed to hypoglycaemia due to injected insulin. He clearly did not appreciate how extremely rare vomiting is in patients with insulin-induced hypoglycaemia. The autopsy itself did nothing to confirm Dr Harris's conclusion as to the cause of the hypoglycaemia but did exclude pancreatic disease, i.e. an insulinoma. Moreover, there was nothing wrong with the liver apart from non-specific fatty changes.

The brain was not preserved intact. This is regrettable, as it is the only organ that can, under the right conditions, provide incontrovertible evidence of hypoglycaemia as the primary cause of death because of the very characteristic changes it can show. Instead only small blocks of it were taken and preserved for possible later use.

Dr Nathaniel Cary, who is a consultant histopathologist and expert in forensic medicine, carried out his first post-mortem on Nic's body on 13th February and his second – the third autopsy in all – on 15th February. His investigations were undertaken at the specific request of Cambridgeshire Constabulary, which had become involved because of the apparently suspicious circumstances surrounding the onset of Nic's illness. Dr Cary confirmed that the immediate cause of death was adult respiratory distress syndrome

There were no visible signs of a tumour in the pancreas that could have been the source of the insulin that Dr Cary, along with the other doctors involved, had presumed initially to be the cause of Nic's hypoglycaemia and death. He was therefore in *"no doubt that insulin was exogenously administered"* and that *"detailed enquiries should be carried out to establish the circumstances in which this occurred"*.

Given such advice, the police had no alternative but to investigate further. They did so over the next 18 months. Amongst the 160 people the police talked to, and from whom they took written evidence, was Professor Robert Forrest, who, as we have already mentioned, is a distinguished chemical pathologist and now Professor of Medical Toxicology in the University of Sheffield and a deputy coroner. He gave them expert professional advice that supported Dr Cary's view that Nic had died as a result of a fatal injection of insulin and, with Dee the only suspect, she was arrested on suspicion in April 1997 and charged with his murder on 29th January 1998, one day less than a year after it was alleged that she administered the fatal dose. She was released on bail until the conclusion of her trial.

It was only then that her defence team approached me. As already mentioned, I already knew something about the case because of my association with Dr Teale, who became an important witness for the prosecution. Dr Teale had worked, first as my assistant and later as a colleague, in the laboratory I had set up 27 years earlier with a specific interest in investigating the causes of hypoglycaemia. Although no longer concerned in its day-to-day activities, I was still a consultant to it and therefore knew something, but not everything, of what was going on in the laboratory.

In the fax confirming my agreement to act as an expert for the defence I said there was *"little doubt, from the evidence I have seen that the patient* [Nic] *– for that is what he was when I first became aware of him – was suffering from factitious (man-made) insulin-induced hypoglycaemia".*

I had based this preliminary opinion solely on the results of the plasma insulin results that I had seen – which is always a dangerous thing to do without knowing anything about the clinical history. I changed my view as I waded through the massive bundle of clinical case notes that eventually arrived along with a host of personal and expert witness statements. My initial opinion – before I knew the details of the case – was based on the fact that Nic had arrived at Hinchinbrooke Hospital suffering from profound hypoglycaemia and that his plasma insulin was inappropriately high and his C-peptide undetectably low. I thought the most likely explanation was that he had given himself insulin – though probably not with suicidal intent, since the concentration of insulin actually reported was very low in comparison with those usually found in suicide cases. It was, however, consistent with self-administration of insulin for other reasons – bodybuilding enthusiasts, for example, know that it builds muscle and its use for this purpose was already being advocated in the bodybuilding magazines. However, by the time I had finished reading the contemporaneous clinical notes, I had become convinced that whatever the cause of Nic's hypoglycaemia, it was very unlikely to have been due to self-administered insulin – as the defence had originally suggested – or to have been due to insulin given with murderous intent by his wife Dee, as the prosecution alleged.

I realized that I could not say with any degree of certainty, from the information then available to me, what had caused Nic's hypoglycaemia – and therefore could not be absolutely sure it was not due to insulin. In my first detailed expert witness statement I came down in favour of the suggestion, apparently made by Dr Matsiko, the consultant looking after Nic, that it was secondary to septicaemia. This was the view Dr Matsiko had expressed in Nic's clinical notes before the results of the insulin assay came through but did not repeat in his written witness statements to the court – presumably having been convinced by the argument that Nic's hypoglycaemia was insulin-induced. I, on the other hand, still think it the more likely explanation.

Dr Matsiko, a general physician with extensive experience of dealing with very sick patients, obviously suspected that Nic had septicaemia, though none of the tests capable of proving this suspicion was carried out until too late in the investigation of his illness. When they were carried out, antibiotics had already been given and would have destroyed any laboratory evidence of infection. The medical notes made on the day Nic died went on to say, *"Initial results do not point to an insulin overdose but we are still waiting the results from Guildford. They should arrive in the next week. The need for a possible coroner's case were* [sic] *discussed"* – indicating that the medical staff were already pretty certain that Nic would soon be dead. There is, however, some confusion on this point since the note containing this information was timed at 10.00 pm on 9th February, or some 12 hours after he was pronounced dead.

Dr Matsiko presumably knew that septicaemia or any severe infection can cause hypoglycaemia. Except in the case of malaria, which Nic clearly did not have, infections do not do so by stimulating the body's own insulin secretion. The plasma insulin and C-peptide levels in cases of hypoglycaemia not due to an insulin-secreting tumour, sulphonylurea poisoning or exogenous insulin are ordinarily low or undetectable. If septicaemia was involved – and, remember, Nic suffered from repeated urinary infections caused by his catheter – then the insulin assay results produced by Dr Teale and Mr Hiscutt would have had to have been wrong.

This is not unreasonable, as we know that immunoassay, the technique used in this case to measure insulin, is subject to analytical error, especially in desperately sick patients, although just how badly it can be affected was not fully appreciated at the time. Awareness of this problem has increased hugely since 2000, when Dee's trial ended.

I was probably, with the benefit of hindsight, unwise to place as much emphasis as I did in my written report on the possibility that Nic's hypoglycaemia was due to septicaemia, as I am not, nor have I ever claimed to be, an expert in this field. I should have stressed even more than I did the likelihood that the insulin measured in Nic's blood was an artefact – in other words that the assay result was erroneous. These things happen. I might have been unduly influenced by the fact that the erroneous insulin measurement, if that is what it was, had been made in Guildford by an old colleague. My report let the prosecution assemble an impressive array of experts on septicaemia – but who knew little about hypoglycaemia – to say that I was wrong. I may have been – though I am still unconvinced, 6 years later, as evidence on the importance of infection as a cause of hypoglycaemia accumulates. My views on the accuracy of the insulin assay results, upon which the whole case hinges, were supported by some of the country's leading experts – but only in the Court of Appeal and not at the trial itself.

Dee's trial

Dee's trial lasted 6 weeks. Much of it was spent in pursuing a red herring that had nothing to do with the cause of Nic's hypoglycaemia but was designed to persuade the jury that Dee wanted so desperately to kill her husband that she was prepared to interfere with his hospital treatment.

Apart from insulin-induced hypoglycaemia and septicaemia, both sides virtually ignored other possible causes of hypoglycaemia or the very genuine possibility that the cause would never be found. My first report was sent to the defence team on 17th April 1999. In it I alluded to some of the possible causes of hypoglycaemia along with my reasons for rejecting the insulin hypothesis. This report reached the prosecution 2 days later and caused such consternation that they immediately applied to the court to vacate the trial date, which had, a year earlier, been set for 9th June 1999 (by then already 2½ years after the events). The court granted the prosecution deferment to enable them to muster a counter-argument against my contention that Nic's hypoglycaemia was very unlikely, on the evidence, to have been due to insulin. I argued, instead, that it was due to some other unspecified cause, of which septicaemia seemed the most likely since it had already been considered by the experienced medical staff looking after Nic at the time and seemed to me to explain the facts better than any other. Moreover, in the very improbable event that insulin was involved, it was far more likely to have been administered by Nic himself for body building rather than by someone else.

The case eventually came to trial in Birmingham in June 2000. The prosecution case against Dee was that Nic had suffered from profound hypoglycaemia as a result of an injection of insulin given to him by Dee sometime between early evening of 30th January, when she left to go to the party with her friends from the hospital, and around 7 am when she was on duty in the wards. A further allegation was that whilst Nic was in intensive care, Dee deliberately, on two occasions, tampered with the intravenous infusion pump so that instead of injecting fluid it injected air into his system. This contention was unsupported by the scientific evidence and was dismissed as irrelevant when the case eventually came to the Court of Appeal. Nevertheless it was given lots of attention during the trial itself and cast so much doubt on Dee's integrity that it could not, I think, have failed to influence the jury.

The evidence, such as it was, for this episode came from a junior nurse who claimed that she found air in the tube linking a pump that was infusing fluid into Nic and which should not have been there. Small quantities of air often get into the tube connecting the bag to the patient when an infusion is nearly or completely finished, especially if the bag is not removed or replaced with a new one in time. According to the nurse, this could not have been the case. Experts called by the defence pointed out that even if – as the prosecution alleged – air in the tube was due to

Dee deliberately interfering with the tubing or by switching off the pump it would have been impossible to introduce enough air to have any adverse effect upon the patient. The prosecution's case was that although this was true, a nurse such as Dee would not be expected to know this (see the Noburo Kato case, page 101). It is a popular fallacy that the tiniest amount of air introduced into a vein is deadly. Having attempted to belittle Dee's medical knowledge in this way, the prosecution then alleged that she had sufficient knowledge of insulin action and dosage to support its contention that she had poisoned Nic with it.

The prosecution more or less admitted that, in the absence of any direct evidence of wrongdoing by Dee, their whole case depended upon the validity of the insulin and C-peptide assay results. It was necessary for the results to be correct and to have been correctly interpreted. Moreover, for the prosecution to succeed, it had to satisfy the jury that Nic could not possibly have injected himself with insulin and that Dee did have access to a supply of insulin and sufficient knowledge of its intensity and duration of action to enable her to inject him with it and for him to be found dead in the morning. They did not entertain the possibility that Nic's hypoglycaemia might not have involved insulin at all nor that if Dee's knowledge of insulin was all that good, she would have known that he might well not have been dead by the time help arrived and would be able, on recovery, to say exactly what had happened to him.

Counsel for the prosecution opened their case by acknowledging that there was no known or discernable motive – a fact drawn to the jury's attention by the judge in his summing up and accepted by the Court of Appeal when it came to them 2 years later. This did not prevent the prosecution from implying, at every opportunity during the trial – and producing witnesses to suggest – that the marriage had run into difficulties and that Nic's death would benefit Dee, who stood to inherit his estate, reputedly worth £625,000. This was the amount Nic had been awarded in 1991 in compensation for his accident and was highlighted as the motive in the extensive press coverage of the trial. Together with the implication – never established – that Nic, despite being sexually impotent, was having an affair with a colleague at work, this must have had a powerful effect upon the jury, whatever the judge said in his summing up.

After the prosecution had presented their case, it was the turn of the defence to rebut it. The only medical evidence called – apart from those who dealt with and shattered the spurious charge that Dee had tampered with the drip pump in the intensive care unit – was from Dr Jennian Geddes, a distinguished neuropathologist with a special interest in hypoglycaemic brain damage, and me.

Dr Geddes, for the defence, agreed with Dr Anderson, for the prosecution, that the small pieces of the brain that were available for examination showed incontrovertible evidence of patchy damage due to failure of the blood supply to the brain but that it was impossible to distinguish this from specific damage that might have been caused by hypoglycaemia. This distinction could probably have been made if the whole brain had been available for examination – but it was not.

The first thing that had struck me while reading Nic's clinical notes when I received them was the pattern of the illness described. It was quite unlike what I had been used to seeing in patients with insulin-induced hypoglycaemia – but not unlike that sometimes seen in patients with other natural causes of hypoglycaemia, such as severe infections, septicaemia, alcohol abuse, and liver, kidney and certain types of glandular disease.

First, and of major importance, Nic had vomited. Now although vomiting and hypoglycaemia can and sometimes do coincide – especially in children – it is because they are both a consequence of the same underlying illness. Insulin-induced hypoglycaemia does not induce vomiting (see the Claus von Bulow case, page 26). It is never cited as a symptom in any of the authoritative surveys of this condition published in the primary biomedical journals over the past 80 years, even though nausea is a very common symptom. Even in the days when thousands of schizophrenia patients were given huge doses of insulin to produce profound hypoglycaemic coma lasting many hours, vomiting from hypoglycaemia was almost unknown. When it did occur, and then extremely rarely, it was always during the recovery phase when massive doses of glucose had been dumped in the stomach through a large-bore stomach tube, which might well induce vomiting. However, many physicians wrongly believe that vomiting is a symptom of insulin-induced hypoglycaemia.

There is a good scientific reason for the absence of vomiting in insulin-induced hypoglycaemia. Experiments both in animals and in humans show that insulin-induced hypoglycaemia hastens the passage of food from the stomach to the intestine. This is a regulatory mechanism that ensures that food in the stomach is digested, and the glucose from it is delivered into the bloodstream to restore blood sugar levels to normal as rapidly as possible.

The prosecution experts disputed my evidence on the rarity of vomiting in insulin-induced hypoglycaemia when the case came to court but, as they were not asked to provide documentary evidence to support their assertions, its presence in Nic's case was not given the clinical and legal significance it deserved. It was, moreover, not the sole or even most important reason for thinking that insulin was not the cause of Nic's hypoglycaemia.

Patients with insulin-induced hypoglycaemic coma do not, when they are discovered unconscious, ordinarily suffer from a "squeaky chest". This usually indicates a respiratory tract infection, asthma or even heart failure. The prosecution experts correctly observed that a "squeaky chest" would be exactly what they would expect to find in a patient who had inhaled vomit. There was, however, no evidence to suggest that Nic had done so – apart from the fact that he had vomited when the ambulance crew moved him to the ambulance and that he had a "squeaky chest" when Dr Roberts first examined him.

When insulin produces hypoglycaemia, the body responds by producing a substance called antidiuretic hormone. This hormone helps adrenaline and glucagon to raise the blood glucose by liberating glucose from the liver, but its main function is to inhibit the kidneys from making urine. Thus, the large volume of urine Nic had produced in the night is evidence against the hypothesis that he had been injected with insulin that night. Dee's disposal of the urine in the catheter bag was presented as an attempt by her to remove evidence that she had poisoned him, rather than a reasonable attempt to empty an overfull bag. Again, this assumes a detailed knowledge of physiology, which the prosecution had argued she did not have. Some urine had been collected from Nic after he arrived in hospital and sent to Guildford along with the plasma sample for analysis. No one knew exactly when this urine sample was collected (i.e. whether it was before or after he had been injected with glucose) and this limited its value as evidence. As previously explained, it contained substantial amounts of C-peptide and smaller amounts of insulin – but this could have been because it had been collected after Nic had already been given intravenous glucose, which had stimulated his own pancreas to produce both insulin and, of course, C-peptide.

Another fact that I noted was Nic's plasma potassium level. Insulin-induced hypoglycaemia normally shifts potassium from the blood into the cells of the body and so often produces a low plasma potassium concentration. Nic's plasma potassium was normal, which suggested, again that he had not been injected with insulin.

Contrary to what is found in many patients who have been given doses of insulin large enough to produce profound and fatal hypoglycaemia, Nic's body had no visible needle tracts, although they were looked for diligently at the time of his admission to hospital. It is impossible to say exactly how big a dose of insulin is required to guarantee that it produces a fatal result, but it is probably not less than 1000 units and in someone as overweight as Nic, who would be insulin-resistant, it is probably considerably more. Injecting this amount of insulin, which is the amount contained in 10 ml of solution, using the extremely fine-gauge insulin needles now used by patients to inject themselves and suggested by the prosecution as having been used by Dee to inject him, would take at least a minute. If a wide-gauge needle, bigger than the one discovered by Dr Roberts, was used, it would be quicker but would leave an obvious needle mark and could not therefore be done surreptitiously. It is difficult to imagine that a grown sentient man who is a trained nurse would willingly let even a devoted companion inject him with a massive and fatal dose of insulin. If Dee had overpowered him, he would have had at least 20 minutes before becoming incapable from hypoglycaemia, and we know that he had phone conversations with his mother and one of his brothers after Dee had left the house.

Professor Forrest got round this difficulty in his first witness statement, written before all the toxicology data were available, though not on the witness stand, by saying, mistakenly, that traces of the "date rape" drug flunitrazepam (Rohypnol) had been found in Nic's urine. Its presence could explain how Dee might have injected him with insulin surreptitiously if he was already doped. In the event there was no flunitrazepam in Nic's urine – only some diazepam injected by the ambulance crew to reduce his muscular spasms on his journey to Hinchinbrooke's Hospital. Had Nic been given flunitrazepam before the insulin injection, he would not have been able to have a conversation with both his mother and one of his brothers after Dee had left the house. Furthermore, had he been given a lethal dose of insulin by Dee before she left the house, he would have been unwell in a way that would have been obvious to his mother and brother when he chatted to them on the phone.

In court it was suggested that Dee had injected Nic with insulin whilst he was asleep without waking him by inserting the needle into the lower part of his body, which was insensitive to pain. This is unlikely. Although Nic could not feel pain below the waist, anything that could ordinarily produce pain sparked off involuntary spasms of his leg muscles and woke him up. These spasms made his life a misery and were only partially alleviated by the treatment he was receiving from his doctor.

An important factor in determining the cause of Nic's death was the failure of glucose to improve his level of consciousness once he arrived at hospital. The fact that only a comparatively small amount of glucose was necessary to re-establish and maintain a normal blood glucose level argues powerfully against his hypoglycaemia being due to insulin. Nic's failure to survive despite the comparatively short interval between the latest possible time of injection of insulin and the beginning of treatment for hypoglycaemia also argues against it being the primary cause of his illness. In most proven cases of murder or attempted murder with insulin in which the victim survives long enough to get to hospital, the amounts of glucose necessary to maintain a normal blood glucose are much larger than in Nic's case and almost always lead to recovery. This is equally true for patients who attempt suicide with insulin. They rarely die unless they have been in a coma for 12 hours or more, or have taken alcohol as well as insulin.

The inability of the prosecution to say when the supposedly fatal injection was given created considerable difficulties for the defence. Its effects would be totally different if it had been given before 8.30 pm on the evening of 30th January than if it had been given around 6 am on the morning of 31st. In their judgment the Court of Appeal said (para 89) *"Although the prosecution did not formally concede that the injection could not have been before the appellant* [Dee Winzar] *left the house for the party at about 8.45 pm she could not realistically have injected the deceased before she left for the party"*. They went on, later in their judgment, to say *"we consider it to be so unlikely that the injection was given before 8.45 pm that this possibility can safely be ruled out"*. They did not, however, conclude, what is indisputable, that it would also have been impossible for Dee to have given the injection earlier than around 3 am, after she and her friends, who were with her all evening, had retired to bed. This timing suggests, improbably, that she had surreptitiously crept away from the Newell household immediately after they had gone to sleep and then, equally surreptitiously, returned to give an appearance of getting up at 6 am in time to get to work at 7 am.

Given this worst-case scenario of Dee leaving her friend's house some time after 2 am, driving home and injecting him with insulin around 3 am, Nic would have been in coma for at most 8 hours when he reached Hinchinbrooke Hospital. If Nic's coma were due solely to hypoglycaemia, he would probably have recovered from his coma, partially or completely, when he was given glucose. This might have taken several days but would probably have happened given that he was correctly treated for brain swelling, which occurs in many conditions and not just in hypoglycaemia.

Whilst insulin cannot be ruled out entirely as the primary cause of Nic's hypoglycaemia, it is, on the evidence, very unlikely – the only reason for suspecting it is the result of the insulin and C-peptide assays. These should therefore have been scrutinized very critically.

On the basis of the evidence they had heard and the slant put on it by the prosecution lawyers, the jury convicted Dee of killing her husband by injecting him with insulin – they made their decision in the space of a few hours, although the trial had lasted 6 weeks. The judge had told them that there was no motive for the murder – if murder there had been – but this was certainly not the impression I gained from what I heard in court and from the press coverage, which spoke of Dee's supposed jealousy and avarice.

By the time of the appeal, a lot of new evidence had accumulated on the unreliability of immunoassays under diverse circumstances. Since the whole case against Dee rested on the reliability of the insulin and C-peptide assays, the defence called four new experts who could address this issue. I was not amongst them and was not called by the defence. The prosecution did, however, call some of the same experts to testify as they had at the original trial.

Dr Adel Ismail, the distinguished clinical biochemist from Bradford, one of the new defence experts, introduced the possibility that Nic might have been the victim of the autoimmune insulin syndrome (AIS). I had mentioned this in my original statement but had dismissed it as sufficiently unlikely as not to warrant further consideration. In AIS blood insulin is increased despite low blood glucose levels. The insulin in AIS is, however, largely inactive because it is tightly, though reversibly, bound to antibodies in the blood plasma. They are called auto-antibodies because they are produced within the patient's body against his own insulin as opposed to therapeutic, i.e. exogenous, insulin. Auto-antibodies to insulin rarely produce symptoms of hypoglycaemia but they often interfere with its measurement.

Insulin is released from the pancreas in response to eating in patients with AIS, exactly as it is in healthy subjects. It is rendered temporarily inactive by binding to antibodies present in their blood. As a result, the blood glucose level rises excessively after a meal, stimulating even more insulin secretion than normal. Eventually, when all the carbohydrate in the meal has been absorbed, the blood glucose begins to fall under the influence of the insulin that becomes 'active' as it slowly disassociates from its antibody binding. About 5 or more hours after the meal there may still be sufficient insulin in the circulation – much of it still bound to antibodies – to produce hypoglycaemia. Because the auto-antibodies rarely bind C-peptide to the same extent as insulin, it disappears from the circulation at the normal rate. Consequently hypoglycaemia produced by AIS, like that produced by exogenous insulin, is associated with a high plasma insulin and low C-peptide level.

It is a requirement for the diagnosis of AIS that the blood contain insulin auto-antibodies in addition to insulin itself. It was common ground that neither Dr Teale nor Dr Hiscutt tested Nic's blood for insulin auto-antibodies, which could therefore have been present and might have accounted for the results reported.

The double dilution test used by Dr Teale, and upon which he relied so heavily in his testimony, reduces, but does not completely eliminate, the possibility that insulin-binding auto-antibodies were present in Nic's blood. If Dr Ismail's suggestion of AIS is right, both the insulin and C-peptide results could have been analytically correct – but the interpretation would have been wrong. Nic's hypoglycaemia would indeed have been insulin-induced but the insulin would have come from his own body rather from a vial. None of the experts called by the prosecution to rebut the new evidence would accept that AIS was a realistic explanation for Nic's illness.

The three other new expert witnesses called by the defence at the appeal – Dr Peter Wood, a specialist in endocrine clinical biochemistry from Southampton, Dr Penny Clarke, an internationally recognized expert in insulin measurement from Birmingham, and Professor Kenneth Bagshawe FRS – were all experts in immunoassay technology. Professor Bagshawe, who was one of the pioneers of immunoassay in the UK and a world authority on cancer, gave evidence as to how and why the insulin analysis results used to convict Dee could have been wrong. Professor Bagshawe was the only defence witness at the appeal who was a medical doctor with experience of treating patients suffering from hypoglycaemia. He agreed under cross-examination, exactly as I had done, that insulin could not conclusively be excluded as the cause of Nic's hypoglycaemia, though he thought it unlikely and that the insulin assay results were wrong.

The Court of Appeal decided that the jury would have convicted Dee even if they had heard the new evidence and that consequently the verdict was safe. They did this after hearing from four experts called by Dee's counsel on the unreliability of insulin immunoassays in the forensic situation and their rebuttal by the same experts who had given evidence for the prosecution at the trial, namely Dr Ferner, Professor Forrest, Dr Teale and Mr Hiscutt.

I believe, however, that the three Court of Appeal judges, like the jury, failed to appreciate that although it is impossible to say with certainty what did cause Nic's hypoglycaemia, it is far from certain that it was insulin. The only reason for believing it to be so was the results of the insulin and C-peptide results, which are quite capable of being wrong. Clinically, Nic's condition was unlike that produced by pharmaceutical insulin in so far as this very rarely produces vomiting and is generally reversed by intravenous glucose when coma is of as short a duration as it undoubtedly was. Insulin-induced hypoglycaemia would not be expected to cause such a rapid fall in plasma albumin within 24 hours of the onset of his illness, as it did in Nic's case, whereas septicaemia-induced hypoglycaemia would.

The possibility of the insulin result being erroneous is not as far fetched as it may at first seem. Indeed, the result of an erroneous immunoassay being responsible for a grave injustice had been established in the Claus von Bulow case some 12 years earlier (see page 46).

Other dire consequences of relying too heavily on immunoassays were receiving international exposure in another case at just about the time Dee was being tried. In that case Jennifer Rufer was awarded $16,000,000 dollars compensation (and many other victims lesser amounts in damages) against the manufacturers of certain immunoassay kits and the laboratories that used them.

Jennifer's ordeal had begun when she was 22 years old. She went to the doctor because of irregular bleeding. The doctor took a blood sample for a routine pregnancy test, one of the most common blood tests performed in the USA. The test, made by Abbott Laboratories, one of the largest diagnostics companies in the world, is an immunoassay test for a hormone called human chorionic gonadotropin (hCG). It was performed on several occasions in the clinical laboratories of Washington University Hospital in Seattle.

The test results consistently came back positive, suggesting that Jennifer was pregnant – but she was not. Further tests were done – all came back strongly positive and still she was not pregnant. Now hCG is, for all practical purposes, produced only by the placenta of pregnant women. The only known exception to this is women who have an extremely rare type of gynaecological cancer known as a choriocarcinoma – or, extraordinarily enough, men who have a choriocarcinoma of the testicle. Numerous tests were carried out on Jennifer to find the site of her presumed choriocarcinoma but none was found. Nevertheless, on the basis of repeated and seemingly incontrovertible (but nonetheless erroneous) evidence of increased amounts of hCG in her blood, Jennifer was treated for cancer. The surgery and drugs used to treat this now curable form of cancer do so only at the cost of producing irreversible side effects, including permanent sterility. By the time she was 25 Jennifer was still alive and apparently well, but sterile, and still with high levels of hCG in her blood.

Jennifer was unsurprisingly concerned by this and expressed some doubt about the validity and accuracy of the tests upon which her doctors placed so much reliance. They clearly did not conform to her clinical condition, since not only was she not pregnant but seemed also not to be suffering from cancer. Eventually she came to the notice of an ultra-specialist in the measurement of hCG in blood, a Dr Laurence Cole. He had refined the immunoassay procedures for measuring hCG and he knew what others should have done but clearly did not – namely that under some circumstances immunoassays can give wildly incorrect results even when, as in Jennifer's case, they were apparently corroborated by tests carried out in different laboratories and using reagents supplied by different manufacturers. Dr Cole established, using highly refined and specific techniques, that the levels of hCG in Jennifer's blood were completely normal and probably always had been. It was just that the tests used to measure it were wrong.

Subsequently Dr Cole saw, and continues to see, dozens of young women who have been wrongly diagnosed as a result of erroneous immunoassay results.

A survey that I carried out involving many thousands of immunoassay tests of all kinds and in laboratories throughout the world showed just how common such errors are. It established that immunoassay results, like all other laboratory test results, should only be accepted as correct if they support a clinical diagnosis.

It is of course much easier to carry out confirmatory tests on living patients than on the dead, in whom – as in Nic McCarthy's case – everything depends upon test results obtained using methods that may fall short of the best and most modern state-of-the-art technology. Unfortunately the methods that Mr Hiscutt and even Dr Teale used to measure insulin in this case fell short of this. Immunoassays owe their popularity to a number of characteristics. However, they are exquisitely sensitive and for most purposes sufficiently specific to make them one of the most valuable tools available to clinical scientists. However, they are insufficiently specific, that is they are comparatively poor at identifying a substance, to be used when the nature of that substance is uncertain. They are too susceptible to interference by a large number of seemingly trivial alterations in the conditions under which the test is performed, of which the presence of auto-antibodies mentioned by Dr Ismail is just one. These interfering substances can give erroneously high as well as erroneously low results, which is why immunoassays, although used for screening in sports medicine and cases involving illegal drug use, are insufficiently reliable to depend upon in court. They must be supplemented either by more specific techniques such as mass spectrometry or by methods that use a technique such as chromatography to purify and identify the substance being tested for prior to their measurement by immunoassay.

Dr Teale used the technique known as 'doubling dilutions'. This is essential when measuring high concentrations of a substance by immunoassay and whilst improving specificity does not establish the accuracy of an immunoassay result beyond doubt. Doubling dilutions reveals some errors but can also conceal others. When questioned about it, Dr Teale, with his typical and characteristic graciousness, admitted that he could not be 100% certain that what he measured was insulin but the dilution results meant it was very likely to be insulin. Professor Forrest was inclined to be even more certain that the analytical results were correct, but on less secure grounds than Dr Teale, upon whose results he relied.

An argument, often referred to as that of prior probability, was introduced by Dr Robin Ferner, an eminent expert on the forensic aspects of hypoglycaemia who had earlier given evidence in the case against Maria Whiston (see page 81). This argument is also known to lawyers and to many lay people as Bayesian logic. It is one of the reasons why – because it might prejudice them – previous convictions are not generally brought to the attention of a jury during a trial. In medicine, knowledge of prior probability is essential for interpreting the results of laboratory tests, none of which is ever 100% reliable. For example, a test with 99% accuracy is extremely valuable in confirming a diagnosis that is already 50% certain. It may, however, be completely useless for screening for the same disease if it is rare in the general population. Take, for example, a disease that occurs in only 1 in 100,000 of the population at any one time. If 100,000 people were tested with a procedure that was 99% accurate, roughly 1000 or 1% would give a positive result, of whom only one would actually have the disease. To find that one in the midst of the thousand with positive results would still be like looking for a needle in a haystack. If, however, the test was administered to someone suffering with the classic symptoms of the rare disease, a test with 99% accuracy would be very useful in confirming that the cause of the symptoms was indeed the rare disease suspected.

Turning again to Nic McCarthy's case, as he was undoubtedly suffering from hypoglycaemia when he came into hospital, it was reasonable – though far from conclusive – to assume that this might be due to insulin, which is responsible for about 50% of cases of hypoglycaemia in people who are not diabetic and receiving treatment with insulin or with sulphonylureas. Prior probability was therefore at least 50% in the minds of the clinicians looking after him (and mine until I read the clinical notes).

On the basis of this argument – and given that the positive finding of insulin in Nic's blood was likely to be correct 99 times out of 100 – the prosecution experts thought his hypoglycaemia and coma "must" have been due to excessive insulin action. The insulin could only have got there from one of two sources – from his pancreas or from an injection. If it came from his pancreas, it would, except in AIS, have been accompanied by high levels of C-peptide – which it was not – and if from a vial it would not.

C-peptide measurements are, like those of insulin, made by immunoassay and are just as fallible. The fact that no C-peptide was found could therefore have been due to its destruction in the blood before it was submitted for analysis or it could, just as I am postulating for insulin, have been due to error in the analysis itself. Both types of error are known to occur. However, because my reason for doubting the accuracy of the insulin result in the first place was that the clinical picture did not suggest insulin poisoning and was quite unlike an insulinoma, I did not pursue either of them in my evidence to the court since the result of the C-peptide analysis was exactly what I expected.

I reasoned, as I have said earlier, that both plasma insulin and C-peptide levels in Nic's blood should have been unrecordably low. I could not give any credibility, therefore, to the proposition originally put forward by the defence, and to which I subscribed until I saw the clinical notes, that Nic might have given himself insulin. Surreptitious self-administration of insulin is many times more common than malicious insulin administration with murderous intent. Surprisingly it is almost as common in people who have no legitimate access to insulin as those, such as people with diabetes, who do.

Nic was a bodybuilder, and it was widely known amongst bodybuilders that insulin can be used to enhance muscular development. In 2000, when Nic died, insulin was readily available at any pharmacy for purchase over the counter. It became a prescription-only drug only after Nic's death.

In the days before the trial the defence lawyers considered whether Nic might, for example, have given himself insulin as part of his bodybuilding regimen or even with suicidal intent. The absence of syringes or insulin in his room at the time of his illness reduces, but does not eliminate, the possibility of self-administration. He could have disposed of them discreetly – though I do not think he did – and he would have had plenty of time to do so since insulin takes at least 20 minutes and generally much longer to produce incapacity. This scenario can, in my opinion, be dismissed on medical grounds. The lawyers found it more difficult to do so on the basis that "my client did not do it and if he did he didn't mean to". In other words, Nic would not have given himself insulin with the intention of committing suicide – which everyone who knew him said was impossible – but he may have done so as part of his bodybuilding exercise. It would have to be done surreptitiously, as it would surely never have been countenanced by Dee, who would have appreciated its dangers. Attractive as the suggestion is, I could not go along with it once I was familiar with the clinical story – it just does not fit.

The prior probability theory works only if the diagnostic test is extremely reliable, and even then it can fail, as in the Jennifer Rufer case. There, despite the use of different tests – albeit all relying on exactly the same principles and equally reliable under ordinary test conditions – she and many other women were wrongly diagnosed as having a choriocarcinoma, an extremely rare tumour. The tragedy of Jennifer's unnecessary treatment for a cancer she did not have would not have happened if corroborative evidence had been sought or a more specific test employed. This case emphasizes the axiom that laboratory test results that are inconsistent with the clinical diagnosis should not be trusted until their veracity has been established beyond any doubt.

Dr Teale and I, with some of our colleagues, once published an account of a patient in which we might well have made an incorrect diagnosis of over- instead of under-active thyroid function had we not had the opportunity of seeing the patient and realizing that the immunoassay results were completely at variance with the patient's clinical condition. This led us to undertake far more thorough investigations than would otherwise have been the case and to confirm that the immunoassay results were incorrect due to interference in the assay procedure. We had published our report in 1986, some 14 years before Dee's trial. This, and similar cases published both before and after us, has confirmed me in the view that I expressed in court as forcibly as I could – namely that when there is a divergence between the clinical picture the patient presents and the laboratory results that are supposed to confirm it, it is essential to question the latter's validity.

In Nic's case I called into question the reliability of the insulin immunoassay test even though a close friend and colleague had performed it, but only after I had reviewed the case as a whole. The four defence experts who testified at the appeal agreed with me. The prosecution experts, who believed the immunoassay test was at least 99% reliable, did not agree with me, but none, apart from Dr Teale, had quite as extensive an experience of either hypoglycaemia or the foibles of immunoassay as those of us on the defence side.

Immunoassay tests are extremely reliable when used on otherwise well patients, but whether they always are in very sick ones has never been put to the test. I am even more sceptical about them now than I was at the time of Dee's trial, as a result of further work Dr Teale and I did together on the diagnostic significance of insulin and C-peptide tests in cases of hypoglycaemia, as well as from evidence published in medical journals.

One such article was published around the time Dee was being tried for murder. It relates, once again, like the Jennifer Rufer case, to the reliability of the immunoassay test for hCG. A group of established French scientists and doctors "measured" hCG in 15 seriously ill men admitted to an intensive care unit in Paris. Much to their surprise, 11 of the 15 men had a positive result on at least one occasion with one of the three immunoassay kits used. This, taken out of context, would suggest that they were all suffering from choriocarcinoma, a very rare cancer of the testicle – which was of course most unlikely. Even more interesting was that as the men recovered from their acute illness, the "hCG" in the blood gradually disappeared and the test eventually became negative. The exact cause for this anomalous and totally unexpected falsification of an otherwise reliable test remains unknown. You wonder what would have happened had they measured insulin as well as hCG. I suspect that something similar would have been observed – namely that they would have found falsely high levels. This, I believe, is what happened to Nic McCarthy. The French publication was not, as far as I am aware, referred to at the Court of Appeal hearing, where only some of the many causes for errors in immunoassays – both analytical and interpretative – were explored.

There is one very well documented series of scientific investigations in which the reliability of insulin immunoassay itself came under critical scrutiny. It began with a paper published in 1978 in the *Proceedings of the National Academy of Sciences of the USA*, one of the most prestigious scientific journals in the world, and emanated from an equally prestigious research group. It was reported, based on immunoassay results, that the brain not only contains, but also produces, insulin. This was contrary to universal belief that the pancreas alone of the bodily organs can produce insulin. Not altogether surprisingly, it caused quite a furore. Rosalyn Yalow, the Nobel Laureate who co-invented immunoassay, became involved. Although the dispute grumbled on for several years, it was eventually accepted that the insulin immunoassay tests used by the original research group – renowned for its immunoassay technology – was at fault and that the brain does not contain or produce insulin. The dispute would be resolved much more quickly nowadays by using more specific methods for measuring insulin than were then available. One such technique uses an initial purification step followed by immunoassay to measure the actual amount of insulin present. It was employed more than 20 years ago in several cases of suspected malicious insulin administration and proved beyond doubt that the insulin circulating in the patient's blood was of animal and not human origin. Since 1997, an equally if not more specific method using mass spectroscopy has been available for measuring insulin in blood in some forensic medicine centres. None of these more discriminatory methods was used in Nic's case.

Measurement of insulin in biological fluids has progressed beyond the stage when we must rely upon immunoassay as the final arbiter of specificity and accuracy in forensic cases, though it remains the linchpin of clinical laboratory practice. The academically important dispute about insulin in the brain that occupied many dozens of pages in the world's most prestigious scientific journals had little impact upon the use of insulin immunoassay for diagnosis in humans. This is because, when they are used – and interpreted – properly, immunoassays are invaluable for elucidating the mechanism through which various illnesses cause hypoglycaemia, as well as in the diagnosis of individual cases.

We now know very much more about the nature and causes of hypoglycaemia than before the immunoassay era began – but far from everything. New and unsuspected causes are still being discovered. This is why I conclude now – as I did then – that there is no satisfactory explanation for Nic's hypoglycaemia. Nor am I certain that it was the cause of his death, which was probably a consequence of an undiagnosed illness. I am just surprised that the jury did not experience similar doubts.

I find it equally perplexing that the Court of Appeal concluded that the jury's confidence in Dee's guilt would not have been dented even if they had heard the new evidence on the unreliability of insulin assay results as this was the linchpin upon which their verdict had to be based. I do not think that the introduction by the prosecution of the red herring of air in the infusion pump tubing, the suggestion that Nic was "playing away from home" and of Dee's jealousy, coupled with her desire to get her hands on the compensation money, had as little bearing on the jury's decision as the Court of Appeal judges believed.

Whether this is yet another example of conviction on the basis of flawed expert evidence will have to await the results of an application to the Criminal Cases Review Body, to which it was referred in 2006 by solicitors acting on Dee's behalf[**]. In the meantime, she is serving a minimum of 15 years in prison for a crime that probably never existed and for which she is a victim twice over – once when she lost her husband and once when she was convicted of the murder that never was.

[**]   Michael Field, Freemans Solicitors, 35 Duke Street, London W1U 1LH.

12 Vicki Jensen, USA: a heinous crime

On 7th March 2002, the Court of Appeal of the State of Idaho confirmed the life sentence imposed on Vicki Jensen for the first-degree murder of her husband's mistress, Aleta Ray.

Vicki was a registered nurse. She had married her second husband, Nicolas, in 1993. In July 1999 her husband left her to live with Aleta, the mother of six children, though only her 3-year-old daughter lived with her. Vicki became increasing distraught following her abandonment and plotted to get her husband back by killing his mistress. She first formulated a plan to kill Aleta by kidnapping her, transporting her to the desert and beating her to death. Vicki's parents, who learned of this plan, confronted her and persuaded her to abandon it.

Some time later, however, Vicki resurrected the idea of murdering her rival and eventually killed her by injecting her with a cocktail of insulin and methylamphetamine, a powerful stimulant sometimes used by drug addicts instead of cocaine.

Vicki was suspected of killing Aleta and arrested, though only after several months of intense investigation by the police, and charged with first-degree murder and conspiracy to murder. Her husband was a key witness at her trial and testified that Vicki had, 2 years earlier, while they were still happily married but during a row about child-support maintenance, threatened that she would kill his ex-wife by injecting her with insulin in the same way as the present victim, his mistress.

It emerged that Vicki had paid her 15-year-old niece, Autumn Marie Pauls, and her niece's boyfriend, Mathew Pearson, to assist her in the plot. They all spent the night preceding the murder in Vicki's house, where they rehearsed what they would do the following morning. The plan was that after her husband had left his new home to go to work, Vicki and her accomplices would go to his apartment and gain admission by knocking on the door. This they did.

Once inside the apartment, they overpowered the victim, who was now alone with her 3-year-old daughter. While one of the accomplices held her, Vicki injected her victim intravenously with insulin and methylamphetamine. She then placed the almost empty methylamphetamine container in the victim's handbag with the intention of making the death look like a drug overdose. The niece and boyfriend gave evidence during the trial that the victim had pleaded with Vicki not to inject her with methylamphetamine, as she was allergic to it.

The conspirators stayed for a further hour until they were certain that the victim would not recover from her insulin-induced coma, before quitting the apartment. It was argued by the prosecution that Vicki could at any time up to their departure have reversed the effects of the insulin by giving the victim sugar, but chose not to do so. Instead she let the victim's toddler watch her mother die alone in the apartment. A fixed life sentence was arrived at as a result of plea-bargaining against an original call for the death penalty, which, in view of the heinousness of the crime and the overwhelming evidence of wrongdoing, the prosecution would probably have obtained.

The Court of Appeals of the State of Idaho dismissed Vicki's appeal for a reduction of sentence, citing the egregious nature of her crime in allowing the victim's 3-year-old child witness her mother's lingering death. Mathew Pearson and Autumn Pauls were both sentenced to life imprisonment, to serve a minimum of 15 and 12 years, respectively.

13 Colin Bouwer, New Zealand: Professor of Psychiatry and murderer

I first heard of Colin Bouwer on 4th March 2001 when I received an email from someone who introduced himself as Detective Sergeant Brett Roberts of Dunedin, New Zealand. The story he told was a fascinating one. Nine months earlier he had arrested Colin Bouwer, who was Head of the Department of Psychiatry in Otago Medical School in Dunedin, on a charge of murdering his wife. During the 3 months preceding his wife's death Colin had written false prescriptions for a long list of drugs, including insulin, which would not ordinarily be prescribed by a psychiatrist except possibly for his own use. The police obtained a search warrant and found on Colin's computer a number of emails that suggested he had injected his wife with insulin some 7–12 hours before her death. He had also emailed a number of international hypoglycaemia experts claiming to be a forensic psychiatrist dealing with a 47-year-old woman who had died in her sleep. The questions he posed related to the injection of insulin or the ingestion of sulphonylurea drugs (medicines used to treat diabetes) and the likely problems of establishing them as a cause of hypoglycaemia.

I was not on Colin Bouwer's email list – nor did I know anyone who was. The police had, however, come across my name as the author of a paper entitled 'Murder by insulin' that I had recently published in the *Medico-Legal Journal*. They wondered whether Colin had phoned or written to me. Just in case I might dismiss his email as a hoax, Sergeant Roberts gave me his telephone number, although his email address – @ police.govt.nz – was a bit of a giveaway. Nevertheless, to be on the safe side, I did phone him as well as replying to his email to say that I had never heard of Dr Bouwer and that he had never been in touch.

I thought that was the end of it until I received a telephone call from Anne Stevens, a barrister, on 1st May 2001. She, and leading counsel David More, were defending Colin Bouwer on a charge of killing his wife by injecting her with insulin after weeks of trying to do so with sulphonylureas. They wanted me to review the evidence and express an opinion.

I agreed to do so and promptly received a mass of clinical notes relating to Colin's wife Annette's last illness during November and December 1999 and her death on 5th January 2000. Anne Stevens also sent me witness statements by a number of local experts who had been consulted by the police. By the end of May I had received a letter from David More – the first of many – enclosing more details of the case against their client and asking for my opinion. He told me that the current defence position was that Annette had suffered from hypoglycaemia due to an insulinoma – an insulin-secreting tumour – and that it had been missed both at operation and at post-mortem. An alternative explanation was that she had committed suicide with drugs her husband had stockpiled for his own suicide when it became evident to her that her doctors could

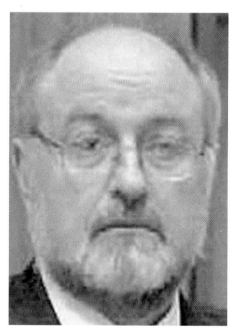

Figure 15 Colin Bouwer.

do no more than they already had done to alleviate her ongoing suffering.

Colin Bouwer was a South African. He was a Consultant Psychiatrist in Dunedin and Professor of Psychiatry in the University of Otago, having left South Africa for New Zealand with his family in 1997. He had already become a pillar of local society and author of several publications. He was apparently happily married to his second wife, Annette, a qualified physiotherapist who was not therefore entirely lacking in medical knowledge. They had a 17-year-old son and a 15-year-old daughter who lived in the family home in Dunedin.

From my point of view, the story proper began at around 6.30 am on the morning of 20th November 1999 when an ambulance arrived at the Bouwer household.

Colin Bouwer had summoned it when he found Annette lying comatose on the bed in her bedroom. The crew confirmed that Annette was in a deep coma (Glasgow Coma Score 3 – the lowest possible when still alive) and, as they had been trained to do on every unconscious patient, measured her blood sugar with a simple point-of-care device (POCD). It was 1.3 mmol/L – easily low enough to account for her coma. They immediately gave her some glucose-containing gel by mouth and then, 5 minutes later, when this failed to have any effect, they injected her with 1 mg of glucagon, a hormone that counteracts insulin by stimulating the liver to release glucose into the circulation.

Thirty minutes later, when the ambulance arrived at the A&E Department* of Dunedin Hospital, Annette's blood sugar level had risen to 5.5 mmol/L, indicating that the glucagon had done its job and overcome her hypoglycaemia. The first doctors to see her said she was sweaty, pale, alert and responsive. They rated her 15 on the Glasgow Coma Scale, which is as good as it gets, and showed that she was fully conscious. She was mildly hypothermic (temperature of 34.7°C), which is common in people who have been hypoglycaemic for any length of time and was so pronounced a feature of Sunny von Bulow's comas (see page 33).

By 7.45 am, Annette's blood sugar level had again fallen to 2.6 mmol/L and, though still fully conscious, she was, to be on the safe side, given a further 25 g of glucose intravenously as a 50% solution. A 5% intravenous glucose drip was also set up. This combination of treatments led to her blood sugar level 10 minutes later being 14.5 mmol/L, which is rather high, and to her urine containing large amounts of glucose.

Annette told the doctors that her health had been declining over the previous 3 weeks and that she had been both very thirsty and very hungry,

---

*   Emergency Room in America.

particularly at night. She had also gained a lot of weight – some 3 kg in the recent past. Other symptoms she complained of were an inability to concentrate, blurring of vision, excessive sweating at night and episodes of poor balance. She denied drinking alcohol to excess or taking any medicines.

Annette was given glucose both by mouth and intravenously and her blood sugar was monitored by a POCD throughout the morning. No formal testing beyond that undertaken on her admission was done in the laboratory until noon, when her blood sugar level had again sunk to 1.2 mmol/L. Although she was still apparently symptom-free, a venous sample of blood was collected and sent to the laboratory to be assayed for glucose, insulin, C-peptide and growth hormone.

For the rest of the day of admission she ate normal meals and continued to receive small doses of glucose intravenously. Despite this, she persistently had "*low blood sugar levels*" within the range 3–3.5 mmol/ L. The rate of glucose infusion was increased to 20 g/hour but even this failed to raise her blood glucose level to normal.

Eventually, at 12.45 am on 21st November, almost 18 hours after she was found comatose, a sample of venous blood was collected and sent to the laboratory for testing for sulphonylureas. Her blood glucose was by this time still only 4–5 mmol/L despite the large amount of glucose she had received.

Analysis of this sample of blood – the results of which were delayed in getting back to the ward – failed to show the presence of any of the five sulphonylurea drugs (tolbutamide, chlorpropamide, glibenclamide, gliclazide and glipizide) available in New Zealand at the time. Surprisingly, no insulin or C-peptide measurements were made on this sample.

Annette continued to receive intravenous glucose at the rate of 15 g/ hour during the whole of 21st November, for much, or all, of 22nd November and seemingly part of 23rd November. At no time, however, was her blood sugar recorded at greater than about 8 mmol/L and for most of the time it was in the range 4–5 mmol/L, i.e. low normal. Her average blood glucose level did not change significantly after the intravenous glucose infusion was stopped. On 23rd November, presumably in the hope of detecting an insulinoma of the pancreas, she underwent a computed tomography (CT) scan of her abdomen, which, not unexpectedly since it rarely does in cases of insulinoma, revealed nothing abnormal.

On 24th November she was interviewed by the Diabetes Nurse Educator, who discussed "*the causes, symptoms and treatment*" of hypoglycaemia with her. She was advised to "*snack*" throughout the day and this she apparently did. The rest of Annette's stay in hospital was uneventful and all investigations, including a CT scan of her skull, were normal.

At the conclusion of this admission Annette was given, on her discharge from hospital, an Advantage meter (a type of instrument used by patients with diabetes to measure their blood glucose) and advised to test her own blood glucose level four times a day before meals as well as during the night, at around 2–3 am, to pick up any nocturnal but asymptomatic hypoglycaemia. She was also advised about the use of Instagel should she develop hypoglycaemia. Instagel is a paste that contains glucose and can be smeared around the inside of the cheeks by a relative or friend should the patient herself be unable to do so. More helpfully, she was given some glucagon, which, unlike Instagel, does work in the unconscious patient but requires someone else to inject it.

Annette was discharged with a provisional diagnosis of hypoglycaemia due to an unknown cause but probably an insulinoma. A follow-up appointment was made for her to see Dr Andrew Bowers, the consultant physician who was looking after her, in 2 weeks' time, by when he would have received the insulin and C-peptide results from the laboratory in another hospital to which they had been sent for analysis.

Just before she was discharged, Annette was tested to rule out adrenocortical insufficiency – a rare but important glandular cause of hypoglycaemia – but in which plasma insulin and C-peptide levels are both low. In Annette's case, when the results on the only sample in which they were measured were eventually received, the concentrations of insulin and C-peptide were both inappropriately high for someone whose blood glucose concentrations was low. This combination occurs, for all practical purposes, in only three situations: a benign tumour of the insulin-secreting tissues of the pancreas (i.e. an insulinoma); a condition resembling it in which all of the islets are affected, though not necessarily morphologically, called non-islet cell hyperinsulinaemic hypoglycaemia (NICHH); and poisoning with one of the sulphonylurea drugs. Sulphonylureas had ostensibly been ruled out by the test carried out 16 hours after she had first come into the hospital and while she still required intravenous glucose to prevent her becoming hypoglycaemic. This left only an insulinoma, or the even rarer condition NICHH, to consider.

Annette was back in hospital just 4 days later. The ambulance crew had again been called by her husband at 6 am on 29th November 1999. They arrived around 6.30 am to find her comatose with a Glasgow Coma Score of 3. The immediate administration of glucagon led her to recover sufficiently to swallow some Instagel. By 7.00 am, her Glasgow Coma Scale reading was 14, which is virtually normal, and, on her arrival at the

A&E Department, her blood glucose was 4.6 mmol/L, which is normal but low for someone who had been given 1 mg of glucagon and glucose by mouth just 40 minutes earlier.

Blood tests made with the Advantage meter during the interval since her first admission showed that on many occasions her blood glucose level had been below 2.5 mmol/L (the level that defines hypoglycaemia) and was sometimes so low as to be incompatible with normal consciousness, suggesting some inaccuracy in making the measurements. At no time, even after meals, did her blood glucose level rise above about 6 mmol/L. This is decidedly abnormal.

Dr Mark Reeves, the first doctor to examine Annette, noted that she was pale and sweaty, and slightly hypothermic with a temperature on admission of 35°C. Her blood sugar level was, however, already normal at 6.1 mmol/L in response to the glucagon she had been given. Dr Reeves collected some venous blood from her and sent it to the laboratory for analysis. In the laboratory the blood glucose level was recorded as 7.4 mmol/L. The plasma insulin level was 299 pmol/L, which is quite appropriate for a blood glucose level of 7.4 mmol/L. Extraordinarily, the plasma C-peptide was not measured on this sample of blood, but might reasonably have been expected also to be normal.

A further venous blood sample, collected at 9.20 am, after Annette had been taken to the wards, was analysed and contained C-peptide at a concentration of 1390 pmol/L, which is high but difficult to interpret since the blood glucose and insulin concentrations were not measured on that particular sample.

Soon after admission on 29th November 1999, Annette was given an intravenous infusion of glucose at the relatively rapid rate of 15 g/hour. This was continued with the addition, from 2nd December, of diazoxide, a drug that blocks the secretion of insulin by the pancreas, especially when it is due to sulphonylurea stimulation. She remained on diazoxide until 10th December, when the dose was temporarily halved before being restored to its original level because of her continuing low blood glucose levels.

Throughout the whole of this time, Annette's blood glucose levels were monitored by frequent bedside (POCD) measurements and were consistently low, often falling below the critical level for diagnosis of hypoglycaemia of 2.5 mmol/L, but no further insulin, C-peptide or pro-insulin measurements were made.

On 1st December, before she was given diazoxide and after discussion with the radiologist, Dr Morrison, Annette had undergone an arterial (calcium) stimulation test. This is a very sophisticated test available only in leading medical institutions even today, let alone in 1999, and is designed to localize an insulin-secreting tumour of the pancreas, which Annette was strongly suspected of suffering from.

In his case notes Dr Morrison described the test as *"routine: no problem"*. His report issued on 2nd December 1999 explained the procedure and said that, *"Following injection* [of calcium gluconate] *into the gastroduodenal artery the blood sugar level dropped from 6 to 1.6 mmol/L"*. This suggests that the calcium injection had caused a large release of insulin, sufficient in fact to lower the blood glucose concentration very substantially, which would not have been expected if the insulin-secreting beta-cells in her pancreas were normal.

In the calcium infusion test blood samples are collected from the hepatic vein (i.e. the one returning blood from the liver to the heart) through a very fine plastic tube, which is inserted into a vein in the groin and threaded up into the hepatic vein under radiological control. This, like the manœuvre required to inject calcium into the various arteries supplying the pancreas with blood, is complicated and depends upon the skills of an interventional radiologist. At the time of Annette's test there were very few units in the world capable of doing it. It is ironic, therefore, that blood collected during the test had to be sent away to a laboratory in Canterbury, New Zealand, for insulin analysis, which was, by 1999, considered routine in many hospital laboratories. To their credit, the Canterbury Laboratory treated the samples as urgent and reported the results almost by return.

The analyses showed that plasma insulin levels in the hepatic vein did not rise after calcium was injected into the artery that supplies the liver with blood – which was only to be expected. What was not expected was that the concentration of insulin in the hepatic vein rose at least twofold after injection of calcium into each of the arteries supplying the pancreas with blood. None of the doctors consulted had ever seen or even heard of a similar result before, and mistakenly interpreted it as indicating an insulin-secreting tumour in the tail of the pancreas. Typically, however, in this condition, a rise in plasma insulin occurs only after the artery supplying the tail of the pancreas has been injected and not when either of the other two arteries supplying the rest of the pancreas are injected.

Annette's diazoxide therapy began the next day and the nursing staff were instructed to monitor her blood pressure as its main clinical use is not to control blood glucose but to lower the blood pressure – which it does only poorly.

Even though she was receiving large doses of glucose intravenously, eating normally and getting diazoxide therapy, Annette's blood glucose level remained low during the whole of her remaining time in hospital. On 5th December, for example, she was described in her clinical notes as "*feeling well*" until 8.00 pm. Her blood sugar level had by this time dropped to 2.9 mmol/L and she became unwell, shaky, dazed and unsteady on her feet. She recovered when given a sugary drink.

Next day Annette was described as being very upset and saying she thought the medication was supposed to help. Later she saw Dr Bowers, the consultant looking after her, who wrote in his notes that Annette, "*feels negative towards medication: she had a hypoglycaemic episode yesterday when her blood glucose was 2.9 mmol/L*". Dr Bowers explained to Annette how diazoxide treatment worked and its function in her case. He also discussed with her the possible need for surgical removal of the insulin-secreting tumour of the pancreas she was believed to have or, if they failed to find one, the effects of partial removal of the pancreas.

Dr Bowers, Dr Patrick Manning, the consultant endocrinologist, and Dr Thomas Elliott, a consultant surgeon, having agreed that the results were most consistent with an insulinoma in the tail of the pancreas, scheduled her for surgery on Monday 13th December. They appeared not to be aware of just how uncharacteristic of a solitary insulinoma the calcium infusion test result was. The anaesthetist consulted by Dr Bowers suggested that for 24 hours prior to surgery Annette should be treated with octreotide (Sandostatin) rather than diazoxide. Octreotide is far more potent than diazoxide for inhibiting insulin secretion. It suffers from the disadvantage that it can only be administered by injection, which limits its usefulness for the treatment of hypoglycaemia caused by an insulin-secreting tumour.

Later that same day Dr Manning told Dr Bowers of his concerns about the results of the calcium stimulation test, which were somewhat unusual. He had discussed them with Professor Halliday of Auckland, an authority on this still novel procedure, who had agreed that Dr Elliott, the surgeon, should remove two-thirds or more of the pancreas if he could not find a solitary tumour. Not altogether surprisingly, Annette was described as "*very anxious and upset*" prior to the operation, which went ahead as scheduled on 13th December. The operation itself and its aftermath were uneventful but Dr Elliot did not find a tumour and therefore proceeded to partial removal of the pancreas in the hope that the bit removed might contain a tumour too small to feel during operation but big enough to produce hypoglycaemia and see under the microscope. Dr Elliot did find a small tumour, a few millimetres in diameter, attached to the surface of the small intestine and removed it. He sent this small tumour and the piece of pancreas and lymph nodes that had been removed with it to the laboratory for examination under the microscope.

Dr Han-Seung Yoon, the hospital pathologist, examined stained slices of the pancreas with a microscope but found no evidence of tumour in it or in the lymph nodes Dr Elliott had removed. He described the small nodule attached to the small intestine as a *"carcinoid tumour consistent with an insulinoma"*. Insulinomas can, extremely rarely, develop outside the pancreas, so here was a possible explanation for Annette's hypoglycaemia. Subsequent examination using a more sophisticated immunostaining technique showed, however, that this particular carcinoid did not contain or secrete insulin. It was therefore not an insulinoma and the mystery remained unresolved.

Annette recovered uneventfully from the operation and her blood glucose level over the next few days was neither too high (above 10 mmol/L) nor too low (below 3.0 mmol/L). She was, however, still on octreotide, as one of its additional actions is to reduce the risk of damage from pancreatic secretions leaking from the cut end of the pancreas after surgery.

On 17th December, 4 days after surgery, Annette was described as *"feeling a little bit unwell"* but her blood sugar was normal at 4.5 mmol/ L. At 10.45 pm that evening she felt slightly light-headed even though her blood sugar levels had been normal at 6 pm and at 9.30 pm.

Octreotide treatment was stopped on 20th December and the glucose infusion discontinued for the first time since her admission. Next day at 10 pm her blood sugar was once again low (3.3 mmol/L), having been normal (5.8 mmol/L) only 4 hours earlier. She ate some food but her blood sugar level rose only very modestly to 4.6 mmol/L, which is less than would be expected if everything was working normally.

Annette was, not surprisingly, even more disconcerted by these low blood sugar levels than she had been previously and was described in the clinical notes as being *"devastated"* by them. Next morning, 22nd December, the medical registrar wrote in her notes that Annette had suffered from symptomatic hypoglycaemia during the night and was quite exhausted by the hypoglycaemic episodes she was experiencing. He described that her blood glucose level had fallen as low as 2.1 mmol/ L the day before but had risen to 4.1 mmol/L by 6 am that morning.

Dr Manning was rather sceptical and queried whether Annette really was still having hypoglycaemic episodes, as up until now the low blood glucose levels had been found only in capillary blood using a self-monitoring device rather than on venous blood measured in the laboratory. He suggested that she should undergo a formal fast-test the following day. This would involve her going without breakfast and having nothing to eat or drink except water over the next 36 hours. The staff were instructed to collect blood for plasma C-peptide and insulin measurements only if her blood glucose fell to less than 2.5 mmol/L. In the event her blood sugar levels remained normal, at between 4.7 and 5.6 mmol/L, during the whole of this period and so no tests for insulin and C-peptide were done.

Because she had not become hypoglycaemic during the fast, Annette was discharged home on Christmas Eve. She was advised that if she experienced any further hypoglycaemic episodes, she should take some sugar by mouth immediately or, if she was unable to swallow, get someone – most probably her husband – to give her an intramuscular injection of glucagon and to take her to A&E without delay. She was instructed to continue monitoring her blood glucose level by pricking her finger and using the POCD as she had been instructed and to report back to the hospital if her blood sugar was low even if she did not have symptoms.

Annette was not prescribed diazoxide or octreotide but went home with a prescription for Creon (a pancreatic enzyme (pancreatin) preparation to assist her digestion since two-thirds of her pancreas had been removed), paracetamol for pain relief and penicillin to prevent the wound becoming infected. It is unclear just how much her husband Colin was involved in the discharge process and the discussions that took place on what should be done if she did become hypoglycaemic at home.

On 2nd January 2000 Colin contacted Dr Manning, who was standing in for Dr Bowers, to say that his wife was not well and that her blood sugar levels were consistently low. He said they were generally between 2.5 and 3.0 mmol/L and that Annette had brief periods of slurred speech and unsteadiness on her feet. He was not unduly concerned, however, because he said that Annette had been told that a blood glucose level as low as 2.5 mmol/L did occasionally occur in healthy individuals – though who, if anyone, would have given such bad advice was never revealed.

On the afternoon of 4th January Colin collected a venous blood sample from Annette and took it to the hospital laboratory for glucose, insulin and C-peptide assay. The blood glucose level was so low, 1.7 mmol/L, that the analyst after checking it for accuracy phoned out the result to the phone number given on the request form as any competent laboratory worker would. He later testified that the specimen he had received was grossly haemolysed and quite unsuitable for the insulin and C-peptide assays that had also been requested. He asked that a further sample be sent – but it never came, as, by next morning, Annette was dead. Consequently the exact cause of her hypoglycaemia at 4.30 pm on 4th January was never established and could only be inferred from what was found at post-mortem.

Colin found Annette dead in bed on the morning of 5th January. She had apparently been dead for some time, though exactly how long was never established. He immediately phoned Dr Bowers, who called round to the house straight away. He confirmed that Annette was dead and that she had apparently vomited. He observed traces of Instagel around her lips, suggesting that someone had tried to resuscitate her, and expressed his willingness to sign a death certificate to the effect that she had died from hypoglycaemia, probably from an insulinoma that had been missed and therefore left behind after the operation. Before doing so, however, and because he had not seen Annette for more than a couple of weeks, he spoke to the coroner, who indicated that he would be satisfied with just a regular hospital post-mortem rather than a forensic one.

At this stage everyone assumed that, despite their best efforts, the surgeons had failed to find a small insulinoma that would undoubtedly be found at post-mortem. Dr Yoon, the Consultant Pathologist in Dunedin Hospital and Associate Professor in the University of Otago, carried out an autopsy on the morning of Annette's death, 5th January. He described the body as that of a middle-aged woman who bore a large bruise at the flexure of the left elbow that contained five needle marks, presumably where Colin had collected blood from Annette the previous day. There was a further needle mark in the flexure of the right elbow.

Her right lung weighed almost twice as much as the left and showed early changes suggesting that Annette had suffered pneumonia from breathing in something noxious, probably the vomit noticed by Dr Bowers. The pericardial space, a virtual cavity that surrounds the heart but which is normally empty, contained 88 ml of fluid. The heart itself appeared to be normal to the naked eye, but examination in the laboratory revealed focal muscle degeneration and patchy inflammation of both the lining of the heart and the heart muscle itself.

The liver showed changes consistent with heart failure, but apart from fat necrosis surrounding the pancreas, which was probably due to her recent surgery, Dr Yoon found nothing else abnormal. He described the brain, which weighed 1386 g, as *"normal"* but did not preserve it intact for later neuropathological examination, as perhaps he should have done in someone who was purported to have died from hypoglycaemia.

He found no evidence of the ventriculo-peritoneal shunt that Colin had told the doctors Annette had been given a few years earlier and which, it was later discovered, was simply an invention of Colin's – it subsequently emerged that Colin was a fantasist and liar on a grand scale. A ventriculo-peritoneal shunt is a tube linking the cavities of the brain to those of the abdomen, and its insertion is a major surgical procedure used to relieve excessive pressure on the brain from accumulation of fluid in it as a result of disease. It could not possibly be overlooked at autopsy by anyone with the appropriate skill.

In the course of the autopsy Dr Yoon collected blood and urine for analysis. He also took a sample of vitreous humour (liquid from the eyeball) to measure its glucose concentration. His initial conclusion, made on the basis of his post-mortem examination of the body and laboratory examination of the tissues he had removed, was that Annette had neither an insulinoma nor pancreatic beta-cell hyperplasia. The latter is an even rarer condition than insulinoma and one in which all of the insulin-secreting cells of the pancreas are abnormal, unlike in insulinoma, when they are localized to a small or tiny tumour the size of a pea or less. Dr Yoon concluded that the abnormalities he had found in Annette's body were most likely due to insulin overdose and not to any abnormality of her own insulin-secreting cells, which he described as normal.

Later, after the opinions of more experienced endocrine pathologists had been sought, Dr Yoon changed his mind and agreed with the opinion expressed by Professor Ian Holdaway, an eminent endocrinologist from Auckland, that Annette's pancreas showed evidence of islet hyperplasia. This is a condition, recognized by examination under the microscope, in which the islets of Langerhans – the tiny packets of specialized cells that secrete insulin and glucagon and are scattered throughout the whole of the pancreas – are uniformly enlarged. Whether Annette did or did not have islet hyperplasia and the differing interpretations put on it figured prominently in the evidence the experts called by the prosecution and by the defence gave on the witness stand.

Annette had alleged, whilst she was in hospital, that she was being poisoned, and so by the time Dr Yoon had finished the naked-eye autopsy and found nothing to account for her death, he decided to discuss the matter with the police. Later that day the police arranged for a forensic post-mortem examination to be conducted by John Blennerhassett, Emeritus Professor of Pathology in the University of Otago in Dunedin on the afternoon of 7th January 2000. During this further examination Professor Blennerhassett found a small benign tumour, 15 mm in diameter, in the tissues in the middle of the chest that had previously been overlooked. He described it as a thymoma. Immuno-histochemical examination confirmed that it, like the small carcinoid removed at operation, did not contain or secrete insulin.

Professor Blennerhassett also noted that Annette's skull was normal and did not contain the holes in it that were required had she really had the ventricular shunt that Colin – for a reason that was never explained – claimed she did. Professor Blennerhassett, like Dr Yoon who later changed his mind, found no evidence of pancreatic islet cell hyperplasia.

Blood samples collected at autopsy by both Dr Yoon and Professor Blennerhassett were sent to Dr Heenan, a toxicologist who, using state-of-the-art technology that was far more sophisticated than that used on Annette's blood whilst she was still alive, found a host of drugs that should not have been there – most of them not ordinarily available except on prescription.

Amongst the drugs found were two different sulphonylureas, glibenclamide and glipizide, both present at concentrations that were within or only slightly above those normally found in diabetic patients treated with them. Metformin, another drug that is used to treat diabetes but which, unlike the sulphonylureas, does not stimulate insulin secretion or cause hypoglycaemia when used alone, was also present at an unbelievably high concentration. Although the original report was shown to contain a transcription error, the concentration of metformin was nevertheless more than five times the maximum level expected in someone receiving legitimate treatment with it.

Also present in Annette's blood was the tranquillizer clonazepam and its major breakdown product, 7-aminoclonezepam. They were present in all of the blood samples sent for analysis by both pathologists and were again several times higher than the therapeutic level, but for some mysterious reasons their concentrations were very different in the samples collected by Dr Yoon and by Professor Blennerhassett.

An antidepressant drug, citalopram, was also found in the post-mortem blood samples. It was subsequently found in the sample of blood that Colin had collected from Annette on the afternoon just before her death, as were glibenclamide and glipizide – but at lower and higher concentrations, respectively, than in the post-mortem blood. This is not altogether surprising, as it is now well known that drug levels in post-mortem blood are often a very poor indicator of their concentration in blood during life.

However, since the sample of blood Colin had collected also had a low blood glucose concentration, it is impossible to escape the conclusion that this was due in part at least, and probably entirely, to the two sulphonylurea drugs acting in concert.

Examination of the stomach contents removed at autopsy showed traces of glibenclamide, glipizide and citalopram. Their concentrations were consistent with those in the blood itself, suggesting that almost all the dose had been absorbed by the time Annette had died. In other words, some considerable time, at least several hours, had elapsed between the times she had last taken the drugs and her death.

By now there could be little doubt that Annette had not died naturally, as Dr Bowers had originally assumed, but was poisoned. The search was on for who was responsible. Had she taken the drugs deliberately because life had become intolerable as a result of the hypoglycaemia that the doctors seemed quite unable to do anything about? Or had Colin systematically poisoned her over the last month or so of her life? The police started an investigation, and 9 months later Colin was on trial on a charge of murdering his wife.

The police investigation soon established a possible motive. Colin was in the midst of a passionate love affair with Dr Anne Walshe, one of his consultant colleagues in the Department of Psychiatry and Psychological Medicine in the University of Otago. She had become Colin's lover following their attendance at a conference in Copenhagen and just a few weeks before he began writing prescriptions for fictitious patients. The first prescription for glibenclamide, a sulphonylurea, was dispensed on 16th November, 4 days before Annette's first hypoglycaemic coma. The last of no less than 11 prescriptions traced to Colin was dispensed at 4 pm on 4th January 2000, just 30 minutes before he took blood from Annette for analysis and sent it to the laboratory. That prescription was the only one to include insulin.

There was no evidence that Anne Walshe was involved with, or knew about, Colin's prescription writing or his subsequent behaviour. The torrid nature of their affair was uncovered when the police looked at Colin's outgoing emails and found some very flowery words of devotion. Anne, for her part, was undoubtedly equally devoted to him, as her daily attendance in court throughout his 6-week trial and her emails confirmed.

Among the things the police discovered in the Bouwer household was a hoard of antidiabetic drugs, including glibenclamide, glipizide and metformin, which would not ordinarily be expected in a psychiatrist's home unless he or a member of his family suffered from type 2 diabetes. Even so, the quantities found were truly enormous by any standards and represented the fruits of the prescriptions that Bouwer had made out in the name of fictitious patients during the 2 months preceding Annette's death. Much was made of the fact that Colin had, when he was first asked about it soon after Annette's first admission to hospital, vehemently denied the possibility that she could have had access to sulphonylureas. To back up his assertion, he claimed to have searched the house and found none.

Research into Colin's background revealed him to be a fantasist of Baron Münchausen proportions. He described himself as having been tortured by the secret police because of his association with the African National Congress (ANC) during the apartheid regime. As a result, he said, he had lost a testicle as well as being subjected to electrical torture. This was untrue, but there was documentary evidence that the South

African Health Professions Council had proclaimed him an impaired doctor because of his addiction to pethidine, a morphine-like painkiller, prior to his departure for New Zealand. His credibility as an upright member of the medical fraternity after he arrived in New Zealand was further dented by the discovery of at least two women patients who claimed to have had sex with him because, as they informed the authorities, he said he had not had sex with his wife for a long time as she had cancer. This was either fantasy or a deliberate lie, as Annette had never had cancer.

My involvement was confined to examining the medical aspects of the case, which were difficult to disentangle from the non-medical, and to express an opinion on them. The medical evidence was of course central to the whole affair. If, as the defence contended, Annette's illness was genuine and happened to coincide with her husband's own planned suicide with hypoglycaemia-inducing drugs – which she discovered only after her final discharge from hospital and used to end her life – the case against him should fail, despite the undoubtedly very strong circumstantial evidence against him.

Annette had undoubtedly suffered from intractable hypoglycaemia throughout the last 6 weeks of her life. According to Colin's lawyer, there was evidence that Dr Geary, the Assistant Dean of the medical school where Colin worked, had suggested, during a casual conversation with Colin 2 months earlier in September 1999, that Annette might have an insulinoma to explain her symptoms rather than the brain tumour that Colin himself said he suspected. No one of course knew at that stage just what a fantasist and liar Colin was, as this only really emerged in the period leading up to his trial. Colin's conversation with Dr Geary was construed as preparatory to what he proposed to do and designed to divert suspicion away from the possibility that Annette's hypoglycaemia was sulphonylurea-induced.

Whatever the motivation for this conversation, there is no doubt that Colin persuaded Annette to have a blood test on 15th November 1999, which showed that everything tested for was normal. The blood test was carried out just 1 day before Colin wrote his first prescription for glibenclamide and only 5 days before Annette had her first hypoglycaemic coma. With hindsight, Annette's hypoglycaemia was inadequately investigated, and the technology used was inadequate in some respects and over the top in others. The failures included not collecting and preserving sufficient blood to undertake a sulphonylurea assay until at least 18 hours after she was first diagnosed with hypoglycaemia, and using a test so insensitive that it could only detect massive overdosing. Dr Bowers did not know this, however, as presumably the analyst never told him, and because the negative test supported Colin's assertion that there were no sulphonylureas in the house – the possibility that Annette's hypoglycaemia was factitious, and caused by these drugs, was dismissed from further consideration.

Professor Evan Begg, the pharmacologist consulted by the prosecution, described the lower limit of sensitivity of the assay used to measure sulphonylureas in Annette's blood sample when she first came into hospital suffering from hypoglycaemia as 176 μg/L, and would only have been capable of detecting a suicidally large dose of sulphonylureas. This assay was 300 times less sensitive than the immunoassay in use in my own laboratory at that time, which could detect as little as 0.5 μg/L. This is sensitive enough to detect sulphonylureas if they are present and responsible for a patient's hypoglycaemia, however long after they have been taken.

Analysis of the last specimen of blood collected from Annette by Colin on the afternoon of her death established that sulphonylureas were – at least on that occasion – associated with her hypoglycaemia, and then only after they had been found in the post-mortem specimens of blood. Although the temptation to attribute all of Annette's earlier hypoglycaemic episodes to sulphonylureas is strong, this was not established by evidence – only by inference.

In retrospect, neither the original sulphonylurea assay result nor Colin's word should have been relied upon, but as so often happens in cases like this, it is easy to be wise after the event. What is somewhat surprising is that despite the recurrence of her hypoglycaemia in hospital after her doctors had failed to find an insulinoma, they did not suspect surreptitious – perhaps self-administered – sulphonylurea use and ask for another assay.

The intra-arterial calcium infusion test result was to play a key role in the evolution of the case against Colin in court. It was unlike that seen in insulinoma patients, but remarkably like that seen in patients with a diffuse abnormality of the islets of Langerhans, the pancreatic cell clusters within the pancreas that produce insulin, as Dr Ian Holdaway, the Professor of Endocrinology in Auckland, had pointed out to Dr Manning, who had consulted him before the Annette's operation. Islets do not need to appear abnormal under the microscope for them to misbehave in response to calcium as though they were insulinoma cells. Dr Yoon, who had originally dismissed the possibility that Annette's islets were enlarged, subsequently agreed that they were. The increased size of the islets was said to result largely from an increase in the number of glucagon-secreting rather than of insulin-secreting cells. This abnormality, the prosecution alleged, was further evidence of chronic sulphonylurea administration rather than a natural abnormality. This seems inherently unlikely as Annette could not have taken the sulphonylurea drugs for more than 6 weeks, at most, and the scientific evidence that sulphonylureas ever produce islet hypertrophy, however long they have been taken for is flimsy.

Islet enlargement is, however, common in patients harbouring an insulinoma as well as in other conditions not associated with hypoglycaemia. Only very rarely is islet hyperplasia the primary cause of intractable hypoglycaemia; far more commonly it is a coincidental finding at autopsy in patients who never experienced hypoglycaemia during life.

If Colin had indeed been giving Annette sulphonylurea drugs, it is difficult to imagine how he did so whilst she was in hospital – and even at home – as she was known to abhor taking medicines of any kind. Even more mysterious is how he managed to get her to take the cocktail of drugs found in her body at autopsy. This included a huge amount of metformin. The prosecution produced evidence that a pestle and mortar they had found in the Bouwer house had been used to grind up glibenclamide and sulphapyridine – a sulphonamide antibiotic that does not produce hypoglycaemia and is only distantly related to the sulphonylureas that do. A plastic jar also found contained a powdered mixture of glibenclamide and sulphasalazine – another sulphonamide antibiotic, which is converted in the body into sulphapyridine.

Since neither sulphapyridine nor sulphasalazine were found in Annette's body, it is difficult to see the relevance of this discovery. Interestingly, the pestle and mortar did not contain metformin. This is so foul-tasting that it is difficult to imagine how it could have got into Annette's body in as large an amount as was found at autopsy unless she had voluntarily swallowed 30 or more tablets or they had been ground up and put down a tube inserted through her mouth into her stomach. This would only have been possible if she had been rendered unconscious by some drug or other, and there would probably have been signs around her mouth of a forced entry – instead her mouth only showed traces of Instagel, which is an antidote to hypoglycaemia!

The trial itself began in Christchurch in October 2001, nearly 2 years after Annette's death. It attracted international attention and lasted 6 weeks. The prosecution called 155 witnesses, of whom 11 were expert or professional witnesses: the defence called just five witnesses, of whom three, including myself, gave expert testimony. Part of the attraction for the world's media was Colin's tall stories, his larger-than-life Walter Mitty character and the fact that his son, by a previous marriage, was simultaneously undergoing investigation in South Africa for murdering his own wife and for which crime he was convicted in 2003.

At one stage the court was linked by satellite television with South Africa, where the doctors who Colin said had operated on him for carcinoma of the prostate whilst he was on bail denied all knowledge of him. They also showed the court a forged letter on their hospital's headed notepaper, describing his illness and its treatment. Another witness introduced evidence that during a tutorial with his students Colin discussed insulin injection between the toes as a perfect means of committing murder. This bizarre and unrealistic suggestion featured in both the Maria Whiston and Deborah Winzar cases in the UK (see pages 91 and 121). In none of them is there a jot of evidence to support the idea that it was done.

The prosecution's case was that Colin had become enamoured of Anne Walshe in September 1999 and hatched a plan to rid himself of his wife and at the same time collect a large insurance premium on her life. He had systematically poisoned her by giving her drugs that would produce hypoglycaemia and eventually, in sufficient overdose, kill her. When this failed to achieve his objective, he used insulin to finish the job. The defence case was that the prosecution had no direct evidence that, until the last days of her life, drugs were in any way implicated in her illness and that her death was caused by drugs she had taken with suicidal intent after discovering her husband's hoard. There is no doubt that she was very depressed by her continuing illness and may well have found out about Colin's affair with Anne Walshe.

Dr Peter Ellis, an Englishman who had been Director of the Department of Forensic Medicine at Westmead Hospital's Institute of Clinical Pathology and Medical Research in Sydney, Australia, was retained as an expert by the defence. With the benefit of 25 years' experience – during which time he had performed some 7000 autopsies – he said that the post-mortem examination of Annette's body had been of poor quality and incapable of elucidating the cause of her death. Instead it seemed to have been performed to seek an elusive insulinoma that was never found. Dr Ellis was particularly critical of the failure to preserve Annette's brain intact for examination by a neuropathologist who could look for the telltale features that characterize hypoglycaemia. He was, in my opinion, absolutely correct in being sceptical of the abnormalities found in Annette's heart being due to hypoglycaemia and appalled by the failure to collect blood for insulin and C-peptide assay at autopsy, as, without it, any charge of poisoning by insulin could be no more than conjecture. Dr Ellis concluded that there was insufficient evidence to specify the cause of Annette's death.

In my view, although their was strong circumstantial evidence that Annette's two admissions to hospital and the hypoglycaemia she suffered following her discharge on Christmas Eve 1999 were due to sulphonylureas, there was no direct evidence for this, although it could easily have been obtained if her doctors had done the relevant tests. There was also the remote possibility that her earlier episodes of hypoglycaemia were due to underlying natural illness, as the doctors treating her suspected right up to the time of her death. This was undoubtedly associated with, and almost certainly due to, the very large number and amount of drugs she had taken in the 12 hours preceding her death, though whether she had taken them voluntarily, or whether her husband had in some way forced them on her, remained for the jury to decide.

In his summing up, which ran to 44 pages of typescript, the judge pointed out that it was for the jury, not the experts, to decide the facts of the case. This is just as well, as I have always considered it my duty to help the courts by giving them the medical facts of the case, as I understand them, and their scientific interpretation, but not to express an opinion on the wider aspects, including whether I think the accused guilty or not. I was, however, criticized by the judge, who in his summing up said, *"Was it inappropriate for an expert of his* [i.e. my] *standing who has flown halfway round the world, to say that he would not discuss the coincidence that Annette Bouwer had within her body this quantity of sulphonylurea drugs? Was it not, when you think about it, quite essential that he do so?"* I contend that if I had expressed an opinion on this matter – which was certainly within the competence of the court – I could, and probably would, have been accused of abrogating the court's and jury's right and duty to make a decision once I had given them the facts upon which to make it. There was of course no evidence that sulphonylureas were present in Annette's body until she died – the only plasma sulphonylurea test performed having "excluded" the possibility.

The judge admitted that the prosecution had been unable to disprove my suggestion that all of Annette's illnesses up to the last day of her life were consistent with her having an extremely rare primary abnormality of her insulin-secreting cells. The original opinion expressed by the prosecution witnesses – that Annette did not have islet hyperplasia – was admitted to have been wrong and it was suggested by the prosecution that this was secondary to sulphonylurea administration. My statement that the evidence for this ever happening was miniscule, especially after as short a time as was postulated in this case, was dismissed as fanciful. I never expressed any doubt that Annette's death was associated with, and caused by, the drugs that were found in her body at post-mortem, but I could not be certain, on clinical grounds, that her hypoglycaemia during the previous 6 weeks was due to sulphonylureas, since the evidence just was not there.

The jury must have been influenced by the coincidence of Colin's bout of improper prescription-writing for hypoglycaemia-producing drugs with the onset of Annette's illness, in which hypoglycaemia, normally a rarity, featured so prominently. Much was made by the prosecution of the number and size of the false prescriptions – the first one alone would have been sufficient to kill several people. Why, unless he was completely deranged, would Colin have accumulated sufficient glibenclamide to kill a regiment, and written prescriptions that were so easily traceable to him?

The suggestion was made early in the trial that Annette might not have died from the drugs found in her body at autopsy but from an injection of insulin that Colin had obtained from a pharmacy, for the first time, on the day of Annette's death. It had been mooted that Colin had used it in desperation when the other drugs had failed to kill her. This line was not very actively pursued, however, as the crucial test of measuring the post-mortem blood samples for insulin and C-peptide that would have proved it – or ruled it out – had not been undertaken; presumably through oversight rather than design. The judge did nonetheless refer to this, without stressing it, in his summing up.

The possibility of a motive, demonstrated by defence counsel to be confined to matrimonial freedom, may also have affected the jury, but possibly the most telling point, stressed by the judge in his summing up, was the statement made by Colin to several witnesses, including Annette's mother, that Annette had a terminal illness long before this was considered, but dismissed, by her medical attendants, who never believed it. The judge in his summing up also emphasized that, on the afternoon before she died, Colin phoned his mother-in-law in South Africa to tell her that Annette was dying but not to bother to come to New Zealand, as Annette would be dead by the time she arrived.

Death from hypoglycaemia is always preventable, as the case of Paul Crampton (see page 59) shows, and Colin's implied callousness in not taking Annette to hospital where she could have been given intravenous glucose probably did more to convince the jury of his guilt than the demonstration that he was an inveterate liar, womanizer and fantasist. Annette was, however, a very strong-minded woman and according to the defence resolutely refused to have any further treatment.

Since Colin has continued to maintain his innocence, the truth about Annette's hypoglycaemia will probably never be known. How, if glibenclamide were the cause of her recurrent hypoglycaemia, did it get into her body without her knowledge? She must have taken it before as well as whilst she was in hospital and after the operation. Even more problematical is how she came to have so much and so many drugs in her body at the end of her life unless she had swallowed them voluntarily.

Colin Bouwer's trial in the High Court of New Zealand in Christ Church lasted from 8th October to 19th November 2001. The jury was out for 3 hours and 25 minutes and returned a guilty verdict. On the same day the Royal College of Psychiatrists of Australia and New Zealand revoked Colin's fellowship of the College. On 18th June 2002 The Court of Appeal of New Zealand dismissed an appeal launched on Colin's behalf by David More and Anne Stevens, his defence lawyers. Instead it upheld an appeal by the Solicitor-General to increase the minimum time that Colin should serve in prison from 13 to 15 years of a mandatory life sentence imposed on him by the trial judge on account of the heinousness of his crime.

14 Elaine Robinson, Wales: a bizarre death

Elaine Robinson was only 43 years old when she died on Thursday 14th April 2000. She had been born in Port Talbot, South Wales, on 23rd March 1957, the fifth of eight children and the youngest girl. She attended St Joseph Comprehensive School, where she was educated to A-level standard. After completing A levels she went on to study teacher training in religious education and drama. She married Stephen Robinson, a native of Warrington, in Greater Liverpool in April 1978 and went to live with him. She had two children by him but they separated in the mid 1980s. They became engaged in a hotly disputed custody battle, as a result of which she gained custody of one child, he the other.

Some time later she became involved in a violent relationship with another man in the Manchester area, by whom she gave birth to her third child in 1990. Whilst living in Manchester she had little contact with her family, but in 1991 she returned to live in Port Talbot. By this time, however, she was pregnant with her fourth child and had begun drinking sufficiently heavily to be described as an alcoholic. All of the children were taken into care.

In 1995, when she was 37, Elaine began a relationship with Kevin Johnson and moved into his house in Port Talbot 4 years later. Kevin was 7 years younger than Elaine and was himself a heavy drinker and drug abuser. At the time she died Elaine was regularly drinking about 5 L of cider a day – or more.

On the afternoon before she died, Elaine and Kevin, together with Elaine's best friend Jacky Jones and her boyfriend, Steven O'Keefe, were drinking cider at Kevin's house. Around 5 pm, Steven left the party to visit his mother, and a mutual friend, Chris Andrews, arrived. Steven rejoined the group at about 7.15 pm and found that Chris had left and the other three were asleep. They soon woke up and, in Steven's words they again *"all started drinking cider together"*. Steven did not notice anything out of the ordinary during the rest of the evening but said later that when they decided to go to bed at about 10.30 pm, Elaine was *"too drunk"* to walk and had to be carried upstairs by him and Kevin. He did not recall that ever happening before.

Next morning, when Kevin woke up and tried to rouse her, Elaine did not respond. His attempts to wake her woke Jacky and Steven, who were asleep in the next bedroom. They came in to find Elaine lying fully clothed on the bed and, according to Steven, *"looking as if she was dead."* Jacky rang 999 and an ambulance arrived at 8.13 am. The two paramedics who made up the ambulance crew assessed the situation and – even although they were unable to find any signs of life – attempted to revive her. They continued to do so for 20 minutes and then set out for Neath Hospital, where Elaine was seen in the A&E Department* a few miles away.

When the ambulance reached the hospital, Elaine was seen straight away by Dr Emma Meredith, an A&E doctor. She noted that Elaine's pupils were dilated and did not respond to light. She had no pulse or audible heart beat, and a heart monitoring machine confirmed that her heart had stopped. Nevertheless she was given glucose, adrenaline and naloxone – an antidote to heroin poisoning – into a vein just in case hypoglycaemia or narcotic poisoning was responsible for her condition. Also, possibly with a coroner's inquest in mind since Elaine's death was both sudden and unexplained, Dr Meredith collected a sample of blood from the main artery in Elaine's thigh before declaring her dead at 9.00 am.

The blood sample Dr Meredith had collected was sent to the chemical pathology laboratory at Neath Hospital for analysis. The blood glucose concentration was only 0.2 mmol/L, or in other words almost zero. However, because no one knew for certain how long Elaine had been dead, this did not necessarily mean that it had been very low whilst she was still alive. The laboratory staff very sensibly saved the rest of the serum in case other tests might be required later.

Elaine's partner Kevin and her friend Jacky did not need hospital treatment but the police surgeon, Dr Ruth Frazer, interviewed both of them later that day. They were both fully conscious and able to tell Dr Frazer what had happened to them.

They described how their friend Chris Andrews had arrived at the party and accepted a drink of cider. Cider was Elaine's favourite tipple, probably because it was cheap, but Chris thought it was rather tame. Soon after Chris arrived, he took a vial of insulin out of his pocket and offered to inject each of the friends with it. He said it would act as a *"pick you up"* or give them a feeling resembling the "speedy" rush they would

---

* Emergency Room in America.

get from amphetamines. However, he needed a syringe. Neither Elaine nor Kevin was a registered drug addict and, though Jacky was, she did not have any syringes with her. Even so, they searched the house and eventually found three syringes in the kitchen that had been left there by a heroin addict who used to live in the house.

Chris drew some insulin into each of the syringes and injected all of the friends in their thighs, and then left about an hour later. Afterwards, all three of them carried on drinking cider but they did not eat anything – or, if they did, they did not remember doing so.

Although neither Jacky nor Kevin appeared to have suffered any very serious or long-lasting adverse effects, Kevin told Dr Frazer that after the injection he felt drowsy, shaky and sweaty. Jacky too said that about 3 hours after she had been injected she began *"to feel sick and shaky"* and remembered *"shaking like a leaf uncontrollably"*. She also recalled that Elaine was *"out of it"* on the settee and looked as though she was drunk. She also remembered Steve and Kevin carrying Elaine up to bed but could not remember when or how many injections she had received. The injections were probably given around 6 pm, as Chris Andrews said he did not stay at Kevin's house for more than an hour.

Dr Frazer's notes, made when she examined them next day, described both Jacky and Kevin as shaking, shivering, tearful and upset. She did not think this was caused by low blood sugar as a result of the insulin injection, but, just to be sure, she took some blood from each of them. She gave the samples to a police office for forensic testing, including measuring their blood glucose. The tests were either overlooked, or their results were for some reason never revealed.

The next expert on the scene was Dr Stephen Leadbeater, a Home Office Forensic Pathologist. He carried out a post-mortem examination on Elaine's body the day after she had died. He described her as a middle-aged woman, 1.67 m tall and weighing 45.1 kg; in other words, she was severely underweight (BMI = 16.17; "normal" = 20–25).

The rest of his anatomical examination revealed no physical disorder that could account for Elaine's death. He thought there might have been a tiny puncture wound on the front of her left thigh but said it was impossible to be sure. He did not remove the tissue from around it for examination in the laboratory.

Elaine's liver weighed 1280 g, which is normal, and when it was examined under a microscope it showed the typical changes of habitual alcohol abuse, which had not yet progressed to permanent cirrhosis.

The samples of blood Dr Leadbeater collected from the main blood vessels of each of her legs contained alcohol, as might have been expected from the events leading up to her death, but only at a very modest concentration of around 40 mg/100 ml, which is half the UK drink-driving limit. This was, it must be remembered, over 12 hours after she had stopped drinking. Between that time and the time of her death, certified as 9 am, Elaine's blood alcohol level would have dropped at a rate of about 15 mg/100 ml of blood/hour. In other words, when she was carried to bed on the night of 13th April, Elaine's blood alcohol concentration would have been in the region of 200 mg/100 ml, which, though high by most people's standards, is not excessively so for a chronic alcoholic and is certainly not fatal. Dr Andrew McKinnon, a forensic scientist at the Metropolitan Laboratory, could not detect even the previous small amount of alcohol in Elaine's blood sample when he tested it 3 months later on 4 July. Instead, he found traces of cannabis and a benzodiazepine-type tranquillizer, though not enough to have killed her. With alcohol poisoning having been ruled out as the cause of her death, suspicion fell on hypoglycaemia resulting from the insulin Chris had given her.

Five days after her death, a sample of Elaine's blood serum was analysed by Dr Rhys John, the distinguished clinical biochemist in charge of the Hormone Reference Laboratory in Cardiff, which did most of the specialist hormone measurements for South Wales. He found that her blood contained 57.7 mU/L (346 pmol/L) of insulin, which would be normal in someone who had just eaten but quite inappropriate for someone who had virtually no glucose in their blood.

Dr John found no C-peptide in Elaine's plasma, which virtually rules out the possibility that the insulin was endogenous. It must have been injected. There was, however, no firm evidence, apart from the absence of C-peptide in her blood, that Elaine had a low blood sugar while she was alive. This is because the only blood glucose measurement was made after Elaine was already dead – and post-mortem blood glucose measurements are known to be unreliable. Nevertheless the fact that two experienced paramedics and a hospital doctor had attempted to revive her suggests that either she was in a state of "suspended animation" – which sometimes happens to patients in profound hypoglycaemic coma and causes them to be wrongly certified as dead – or that she was not long dead when the ambulance crew arrived. If this was so, Elaine's blood glucose concentration of only 0.2 mmol/L assumed much more importance. In any event, it was perfectly consistent with her having died from hypoglycaemia.

For good measure, on 28th April 2000, which was 14 days after Elaine's death, Dr John analysed the contents of a bottle the police had seized from Kevin's house and labelled Human Mixtard. It confirmed that the bottle contained insulin at the expected concentration of around 100 units/ml.

It was at this stage that I was consulted and asked to advise whether Elaine's death could properly be laid at Chris Andrews' door. After all, she was not alone in having been given insulin and neither of the other two had come to any harm.

I read all the evidence and concluded that Elaine's death on the morning of 14th April 2000 was attributable to the injection of insulin she had received on the evening of 13th April but that the exact time of her death was difficult to determine.

I noted that Elaine's plasma insulin level was inappropriately high for someone who had not eaten within the past 2 hours – and all the more so in someone as skinny as she was. A high plasma insulin level, however, does not prove that the low blood sugar level was due to an insulin injection – it might have been an erroneous measurement, as we know can occur. Her low blood glucose, it could be argued, was the result of her malnutrition, alcohol abuse or both. Hypoglycaemia produced by them is associated with low or undetectable C-peptide levels in the blood. This is because hypoglycaemia suppresses C-peptide production in every situation except when it is caused by an insulin-secreting tumour of the pancreas (which is rare) or a sulphonylurea overdose. Neither of these was remotely likely in Elaine's case. I concluded that the evidence from the blood test, combined with the clinical evidence that Elaine was already suffering from hypoglycaemia the previous evening to such an extent that she was thought to be more drunk than any of her friends had ever seen her before, and the history given by her friends, made the case for insulin poisoning almost incontrovertible.

It is impossible to say how much insulin Elaine actually received on that fatal evening, but it may well only have been in the region of 50–100 units. This would not ordinarily be sufficient to kill a healthy well-nourished person but could – and undoubtedly did – kill Elaine.

Why then did she, but not the others, respond so badly to what could only have been a modest overdose of insulin? The amount would not have been expected to kill anyone – even someone as malnourished as Elaine – and certainly not as quickly as it undoubtedly did. The answer is that alcohol and hypoglycaemia go very badly together, as studies of people who attempt suicide with insulin have shown. Indeed, a very high proportion of people who successfully kill themselves with insulin do so only because they have also taken either alcohol or certain prescription drugs.

But could not the alcohol itself have been responsible for Elaine's hypoglycaemia – exactly as it was in Sunny von Bulow's case (see page 42)? This possibility had to be considered, but it was ruled out by two laboratory tests. The first showed that there was a substantial amount of insulin in Elaine's blood, which there would not have been if her hypoglycaemia had been due to alcohol, as this causes hypoglycaemia through an entirely different mechanism. The other test was carried out on a fluid in the eye called vitreous humour. Dr Leadbeater had collected a sample of this at the post-mortem. It revealed a low concentration (200 μmol/L) of a substance called beta-hydroxybutyrate. This occurs at high concentration in the blood and presumably vitreous humour of people who die from alcohol-induced hypoglycaemia but not in those who die from insulin-induced hypoglycaemia.

Strange as it may seem, insulin has been used, probably rarely, by drug abusers for the side effects it regularly produces, and this must have been what motivated Chris Andrews to offer Elaine and her friends "a fix" with insulin. Diabetic patients who have to take insulin consider these effects undesirable, unpleasant and to be avoided if at all possible. The symptoms are accompanied by an adrenaline surge resembling, in some respects, that produced by the intravenous injection of amphetamines. It was presumably with this in mind rather than any evil intent that Chris offered Elaine and her friends some of the insulin – which he had obtained from a diabetic patient for whom it had been legitimately prescribed.

Insulin had been freely available from regular pharmacies without prescription until only a year before Elaine died. It had been put on the prescription-only list because of widespread abuse by bodybuilders, who believed it helped them build up muscles (shades of Nic McCarthy, in whom its use was raised as a possibility but dismissed as fanciful, see page 129).

On the basis of my report, the Crown Prosecution Service felt sufficiently confident to charge Chris Andrews with the manslaughter of Elaine Robertson, to which charge he pleaded guilty on 24th October 2001 at Swansea Crown Court. Three other charges of causing a noxious thing to be taken with intent to endanger life (of Elaine, Kevin and Jacky) were not pursued but ordered to lie on the file. He was sentenced to 2 years in jail.

Despite having pleaded guilty, Chris later appealed against his conviction and sentence. His appeal was based on the contention that insulin is not a noxious substance and that Elaine had been in obvious agreement to the injection. The appeal was heard at the Court of Appeal in London on 21st November 2001. It failed.

The argument in the Court of Appeal boiled down to the exact nature and wording of the charges against Chris Andrews rather than the nature or heinousness of his crime. Clearly he did not intend to kill Elaine but did so by behaving recklessly. My opinion is that the question of Chris's guilt and appeal outcome would have been different had insulin been an over-the-counter drug, which it had been until a year earlier. He would probably have been acquitted of any crime.

Appendix

Background to technical terms

Glucose

Glucose is a simple sugar: this means that it cannot be split into other sugars, as complex sugars, for example sucrose and lactose, can. The only simple sugars of importance to us in our diet are glucose, fructose and galactose. Only glucose occurs in the blood in more than infinitesimal amounts except in disease. Simple sugars are the building blocks from which other dietary carbohydrates are built and the only ones that can be absorbed. Starches, sucrose (or cane sugar) and lactose (or milk sugar) must all be broken down into their constituent simple sugars by enzymes in the gut before they can be absorbed. Once in the blood, fructose (from table sugar and fruit) and galactose (from milk) are removed by the liver before they get into the general circulation. The liver turns them into glycogen, the storage form of glucose, for release into the blood as required. About 60% of the glucose absorbed from a meal passes through the liver and enters the general circulation, from which it is removed by the tissues and used as fuel. About 40% is taken up by the liver and turned into glycogen.

The liver is the only organ in the body that can store glucose and release it back into the blood. It does this as soon as all of the last meal has been absorbed – usually about 3–6 hours after it was eaten unless it was a very large or very small one. The liver also has the capacity to make new glucose from simpler building blocks brought to it in the blood from the other tissues and which are the breakdown products of their own stores of energy. The most important of these building blocks are lactic acid, pyruvic acid, glycerol and alanine. This process is continuous but accelerates enormously during periods of prolonged fasting, although not as rapidly as it does in patients with type 1 diabetes, who cannot make their own insulin.

In the absence of insulin, glucose is unavailable to most of the tissues of the body except the brain. But the brain cannot use glucose as fast as it can be absorbed after a meal or, in patients with type 1 diabetes, as fast as the liver produces it during fasting. Consequently glucose accumulates in the blood and produces the very high blood glucose levels that are characteristic of diabetes.

Because bodily tissues cannot extract glucose and use it as fuel, when no insulin is available they resort to using fats or, more particularly, free fatty acids. These are released from fat stores in adipose tissue when insulin is unavailable and are carried to the tissues, where they are extracted from the circulation and used to supply energy. It is only because we all have substantial amounts of fat in our bodies that we can withstand fasting for many days on end without coming to serious harm, although we may experience severe hunger, which, though unpleasant, is not dangerous.

The liver uses fatty acids brought to it in the blood from body stores in different ways depending upon how much insulin and glucagon are present. When insulin is plentiful the liver stores fats as triglycerides, but when it is lacking it turns them into two closely related substances called ketones. These, like fatty acids, can be used as fuel by tissues such as the heart and muscles, but, unlike fatty acids, they can, under certain circumstances, also be used by the brain.

Blood glucose

The concentration of glucose in the blood, which reflects the total amount of glucose in the body, stays within remarkably narrow limits throughout the day despite the intermittency of its supply in food. It rarely rises above 10 mmol/L (equivalent to about 1.8 g of glucose/L of blood) after the largest meal or falls below 3.5 mmol/L (0.72 g/L) after several days without food. This control is lost when insulin secretion is defective. Too much insulin produces abnormally low glucose levels; too little produces abnormally high ones. High blood glucose levels are associated with diabetes, low blood glucose levels with abnormalities of brain function known as hypoglycaemia or just hypo.

The symptoms produced by hypoglycaemia are due to its effects upon the brain. The brain relies upon a constant and adequate supply of glucose coming to it in the blood in much the same way as it needs oxygen. Just as with lack of oxygen, hypoglycaemia can cause permanent brain damage and death if it persists for long enough. Unlike asphyxia, resulting from restricted supplies of oxygen, the body does have reserves of glucose that it can call upon when the brain is threatened by hypoglycaemia, and there is an extensive and well organized machinery for doing this.

The defence mechanism relies upon the release of several hormones, of which glucagon and adrenaline are the most important, although others, including noradrenaline, cortisol, growth hormone and vasopressin, also play a part. Only when overdosing with insulin is excessive or when for some reason there is no glycogen in the liver do they fail to deliver enough glucose into the circulation to prevent the brain becoming permanently damaged.

No one knows for certain for how long the blood glucose concentration has to be low – and how low it has or be – to produce permanent brain damage. The best estimate I have been able to come up with is based upon clinical observations on patients who have tried to commit suicide with insulin, or have been given it as a treatment for schizophrenia in the past, and upon research undertaken on monkeys. The data suggest that permanent brain damage is likely when the blood glucose concentration remains at less than 1.1 mmol/L for 5 hours or more. Undoubtedly some patients who suffer less severe hypoglycaemia for shorter periods do sustain permanent brain damage, or die, but others have survived unscathed after having been hypoglycaemic for longer.

The shorter the period of severe hypoglycaemia associated with coma the more likely is the patient to recover consciousness immediately (or almost immediately) their blood glucose level is restored to normal with intravenous glucose. All is not lost, however, even when this fails to work. Full recovery can occur up to several days later, providing the blood glucose level is kept within the normal range by intravenous glucose, and raised intracranial pressure due to swelling of the brain (as sometimes occurs) is reduced by appropriate treatment. Almost all patients who are found alive after attempting suicide with insulin recover completely when treated appropriately.

Insulin

Treatment of diabetes with insulin has been commonplace since 1922. Insulin is a polypeptide hormone, or chemical messenger, made only in the beta-cells of the pancreas. These special cells, found nowhere else in the body, are packaged, along with others called alpha-cells, which produce a hormone called glucagon, into tiny organelles know as islets of Langerhans. These are scattered throughout the bulk of the pancreas, which weighs about 100 g (4 oz) and whose main function is to produce the enzymes that enable us to digest food. There are about one million islets, each of which is less than 1 mm (0.04 inch) in diameter, and whose role is to control the blood glucose level within the narrow limits described above. This is no mean task and often goes wrong, especially, but not only, in patients with diabetes.

Insulin and glucagon are both small proteins that once released into the bloodstream are rapidly removed by attaching themselves to the cells where they exert their biological effects. Insulin attaches to almost every type of cell, enabling them to extract glucose from the blood, and, in the case of the liver, prevents it from releasing its stores into the blood. Glucagon, on the other hand, attaches itself only to liver cells and encourages them to release their glucose stores into the blood. In other words, whilst insulin lowers the concentration of glucose in the blood, glucagon raises it.

The release of both of these hormones is regulated in healthy people by the concentration of glucose in the blood. As the concentration rises, after eating a meal, insulin secretion goes up and glucagon secretion goes down. Once all the food has been absorbed, usually after 3–6 hours, the process goes into reverse.

In people with diabetes the beta-cells are unable to produce insulin properly and it must be replaced by injection since, being a protein, it cannot be taken by mouth as it would be digested before it could be absorbed. The cells of the brain do not require insulin to remove glucose from the blood and use it. All other cells do. Overweight people, and those with a condition called insulin resistance, require more insulin to do this than thin people.

Surprisingly, although illnesses due to abnormalities of insulin secretion, especially diabetes, are very common, those due to abnormalities of glucagon are almost unknown and, unlike insulin, it is not essential for life. In the most florid form of diabetes there is an inability to produce any insulin at all, but in most patients some capacity remains.

A very much rarer abnormality of insulin secretion is that produced by tumours or – even more rarely – functional abnormalities of pancreatic beta-cells. In this condition the beta-cells carry on releasing insulin into the blood, even though the blood glucose level is already low, and cause it to fall even lower.

The amount of insulin in the body when it is given by injection cannot be regulated with the same precision as by the healthy pancreas. As a result there is sometimes more insulin in the blood than the body needs and the blood glucose level falls so low that the brain stops working properly. As well as in cases of insulin overdose, this can occur in patients with insulin-secreting tumours and those taking sulphonylurea drugs for the treatment of diabetes or, rarely, in any one of about a 100 other illnesses, in most of which insulin is not involved and blood insulin levels are low.

Donald Steiner, a colleague of Arthur Rubenstein in Chicago, discovered C-peptide in 1967 and showed that it was an essential building block in the manufacture of insulin within the beta-cells of the pancreas. The immediate precursor of insulin, called pro-insulin, is split into two substances – C-peptide and insulin – which are stored in tiny granules within the beta-cells until they are secreted simultaneously into the blood in response to a meal. No one knows exactly what C-peptide does in the body, but it is certainly not the inert substance scientists once believed. Clinicians and forensic scientist use it extensively to distinguish insulin in the blood that came from a bottle – and which contains no C-peptide – from insulin that originated in the pancreas.

Insulin that comes from the pancreas is always accompanied by C-peptide. This can be measured at the same time as insulin, using a similar method. The two results make differentiation of endogenous insulin (i.e. that made in the pancreas) from exogenous or pharmaceutical insulin (i.e. from a bottle) very easy in theory. Once they get into the blood insulin and C-peptide behave very differently from one another and it sometimes happens that a patient's blood can contain, or appears to contain, one without the other. When this anomaly occurs whilst the patient is still alive it is usually possible to resolve the problem by repeating the analyses and doing further tests. This option may not be open in forensic cases such as are described in this book where blood tests are the only evidence of wrongdoing and can lead to miscarriages of justice.

Symptoms of and death from hypoglycaemia

Patients suffer a variety of symptoms as a result of hypoglycaemia. They are usually relatively mild and are easily reversed by eating or drinking something sugary. They are experienced from time to time by every insulin-treated patient with diabetes and usually do not proceed to coma even if left untreated, as the body has such good defences against it. The most common symptoms include anxiety, profuse sweating, a sense of inner trembling, rapid heart beat, tingling in the fingers and around the lips, blurring of vision, and a general feeling of unwellness. They may progress to a state where the patient loses consciousness.

Patients can die from hypoglycaemia – usually from multiorgan failure after a prolonged period of coma – but this is rare. They may, however, die much more abruptly. The mechanism for this is unknown but it is suspected as being due to the sudden rush of adrenaline, released into the blood in response to a rapidly falling blood glucose concentration, triggering an electrical disturbance in the heart. It is thought to be responsible for some of the cases of "found dead in bed", which is the name given to unexplained sudden death occurring, especially in young people, treated with insulin.

In them, as in those who successfully commit suicide with insulin and victims of murder by insulin, an ordinary post-mortem examination fails to reveal an immediate anatomical cause. It is only if the patient survives for several days after he suffered irreversible and permanent damage that the characteristic changes appear in the brain that enable a skilled neuropathologist to make a definitive diagnosis of hypoglycaemic brain damage.

Because glucose disappears from the blood after death, its measurement in a corpse can do no more than establish that the blood glucose level was normal or high – never that it was low – at the time of death. Insulin and C-peptide can be measured in blood collected after death, providing it is possible to obtain serum separated from the red cells. If the red cells have burst, which is called haemolysis, the results will not be valid.

Measurement of insulin and C-peptide in blood

In 1960 two Americans, Solomon Berson and Rosalyn Yalow, invented a method called radioimmunoassay that was sensitive enough to measure the concentration of insulin in the blood of living people. Before that time only very rough estimates were possible and these were obtained using techniques that made them useless for ordinary clinical work though useful for research. With the invention of radioimmunoassay, knowledge of the way the body makes, uses and disposes of insulin increased in leaps and bounds. The method was soon applied to the diagnosis of patients with diabetes but proved disappointing clinically. Insulin measurements add little to the measurement of glucose, which is both much simpler and cheaper. The main use of insulin measurements in the clinic is in helping to determine the cause of hypoglycaemia, only some cases of which are due to insulin. Their usefulness in the diagnosis of hypoglycaemia increased enormously with the discovery of C-peptide and the introduction of a method of measuring it by Arthur Rubenstein and his co-workers in the mid 1970s.

Methods for measuring insulin have changed since Yalow and Berson invented radioimmunoassay, but most still use antibodies. All are open to interference from extraneous substances that can give totally misleading results. The list of causes of 'wrong answers' to insulin (and C-peptide) immunoassay results is quite long, though most are extremely rare. Interference can be overcome by the use of a very sophisticated technique called mass spectrometry, which though introduced for this purpose almost 10 years ago, was not applied in any of the cases described in this book. It has so far never been used in a proven case of murder by insulin. It may not be necessary in most cases, but where doubt exists as to whether what appears to have been measured as insulin really is insulin, mass spectrometry, for example, or other sophisticated methods using a separation techniques should, in my view, be used for a conviction based upon the result to be considered safe.

Glossary

Name (abbreviation)	Comment
Accurate and accuracy	An accurate result is one that is very close to the true answer – the concentration of a substance in a solution, for example. It depends upon both the specificity and the precision of the analysis
Albumin	The most plentiful protein in plasma/serum, with a "half-life" of about 19 days. A rapid fall in concentration over a few days is always due to its leakage from the circulation into the interstial fluid and is characteristic of surgical shock or septicaemia
Antibody	A protein that combines tightly, but usually reversibly, with an antigen, i.e. a substance capable of provoking an antibody response when injected into an animal. Antibodies are the key reagent in all immunoassays. In life antibodies neutralize the biological or toxic effects of an antigen, so that someone can have a lot of antibody-bound insulin in their blood without it having very much effect on their blood sugar
Antisera	Antisera are obtained from animals that have been immunized and contain antibodies (see above). These are specific proteins produced by an animal immunized with a substance and react only with that substance or substances very like it
Barbiturates	A group of drugs used to treat insomnia and which in overdose can cause coma or death. Rarely used nowadays but once a favorite way of committing suicide

Name (abbreviation)	Comment
Benzodiazepines	A group of drugs used to treat anxiety and insomnia. They are tasteless and when added to drinks make people behave recklessly as though they are intoxicated. One of these drugs, Rohypnol (flunitrazepam) has achieved notoriety as the "date-rape" drug, but all benzodiazepines produce similar effects
Body mass index (BMI)	Now a generally accepted measure of "plumpness". It is derived from a formula that takes into account the person's weight and height. Any BMI below 20 is indicative of thinness and may indicate malnutrition
Carcinoid	A tumour with a characterisitc histological appearance and usually found in the gastrointestinal tract. Usually of low or no malignancy. Carcinoids may – though only very rarely – produce various hormones, including insulin
Chorionic gonadotropin ((h)CG)	A protein hormone produced exclusively by the placenta and measured in blood as an early sign of pregancy
Coma	A state of unconsciousness from which the patient cannot be aroused and in which all but the most primitive of reflexes are lost
Diagnosis	Literally an understanding of the patient's illness through a knowledge especially of its cause. Hypoglycaemia is only a partial diagnosis – or description – it only becomes a proper diagnosis when it can be attributed to a cause
Diazoxide	A drug that has the specific property of inhibiting insulin secretion by the beta-cells of the pancreas
Factitious	Intentionally fabricated usually applied to a disease or illness deliberately produced by a patient in order to gain attention. Factitious hypoglycaemia is usally produced by surrepticious self-injection of insulin. Everything the patient tells the doctors about his illness is true except the fact that he is producing it himself. Patient will go to extraordinary lengths to conceal the truth
False negative	The term used in clinical and forensic medicine to describe the exclusion, or dismissing, of a correct diagnosis on the basis of a laboratory result (measurement). A false negative may be caused by a laboratory error but more commonly by incorrect interpretation of an accurate result

Name (abbreviation)	Comment
False positive	The term used in clinical and forensic medicine to describe the making of an incorrect diagnosis on the basis of a laboratory result (measurement). A false positive may be caused by laboratory error but is more commonly due to an incorrect interpretation of an accurate result
Haemolysis	This occurs when the red blood cells burst open, liberating their red pigment, haemoglobin, into the plasma or serum, giving it a pink to dark red colour depending on the number of cells involved. It always occurs after about 24 hours but may occur much quicker, especially if the blood sample is not collected correctly
Histology	Examination of the tissues of the body under the microscope – usually to help make a diagnosis
Histopathologist	A pathologist who specializes in making a diagnosis by examining the tissues of the body and by performing autopsies
Immunoassay	A method for measuring substances that uses an antibody raised in an animal against the substance that is being measured
Insulin	A protein hormone made exclusively by the beta-cells of the pancreas. Insulins differ very slightly depending upon which animal they come from and whether they are synthetically made. This can cause problems when it comes to measuring insulin in blood as insulins behave differently from one another in immunoassays. This is especially true of the new synthetic insulins
Metformin	A medicine used to treat patients with type 2 diabetes but which does not, unlike the sulphonylureas, stimulate insulin secretion and never causes hypoglycaemia
Microgram (µg)	A millionth of a gram
Milligram (mg)	A thousandth of a gram or a millionth of a kilogram
Millimole (mmol)	One thousandth of a mole: a millimole of glucose weighs 180 milligrams and 1 mmol/L = 180 mg glucose/litre
Milliunit (mU)	The unit used to describe the concentration of insulin in 1 litre of blood before it became possible to express it in more precise chemical terms, i.e. as picomoles. 1 mU of insulin/litre of blood is the same as 7 picomoles of insulin/litre of blood

Name (abbreviation)	Comment
Mole (mol)	A sophisticated but very useful way of expressing the amount of a substance. It is used by chemists and physicists and takes into account the fact that molecules have different weights. (For the purist a mole can be defined as the amount of substance that contains as many elementary entities as there are atoms in exactly 0.012 kg of carbon-12. This quantity is known as Avogadro's number and is approximately [sic] $6.02214199 \times 10^{23}$)
Nanogram (ng)	A thousand millionth of a gram
Normal	In statistics "normal" describes the even distribution about the mean in a number of observations of a single entity – plotted on graph paper it produces the typical bell-shaped curve. Often used colloquially as synonymous with healthy. Its use in this context has been replaced in laboratory medicine by the term "reference range"
Neuropathologist	A pathologist who specializes in detailed examination of the brain after death
Octreotide	A drug that inhibits the secretion of a number of protein hormones, including insulin
Pathologist	A scientist, usually one who is medically qualified, who studies the causes of disease. Some pathologists, a minority, undertake autopsies whether for legal (forensic) or medical (clinical) reasons. Most pathologists are involved in research and with the diagnosis and treatment of disease
pH	The most common way of expressing the acidity or concentration of hydrogen ions of something. The scale is a logarithmic one extending from 0 to 14. Absolute neutrality (ultrapure water) is represented by a pH of 7.0000. In healthy people the pH of blood is kept very close to 7.4 or slightly alkaline – a drop to 7.2 indicates the accumulation of many hydrogen ions (increased acidity) and a pH of 7.0 is barely compatible with life
Picogram (pg)	A million millionth of a gram
Picomole (pmol)	A million millionth of a mole: one picomole of insulin weighs 6 nanograms (6 billionths of a gram)

Name (abbreviation)	Comment
Plasma	The fluid in which the red and white cells of the blood are suspended in the body. The fluid remaining after the red cells have been removed to form a blood clot is called serum
Point of care (testing) devices (POCD)	These can be used to measure glucose and other substances in blood at the patient's bedside
Precision	This is a measure of the reproducibility of a method when it is undertaken many times on the same sample. A method that is very precise but not very specific may, in some circumstances, give inaccurate results
Radioimmunoassay (RIA)	The first type of immunoassay to be invented. Other types of immunoassay are now also used but all require at least one and usually more antibodies employed in a variety of different ways
Red blood cells	The tiny packages of haemoglobin that are suspended in the blood plasma and give blood its red colour. Red cells that are larger than "normal" are called macrocytes, those smaller than normal "microcytes"
Sensitivity	This is a measure of the least or smallest amount of a substance that can be distinguished with mathematical confidence from zero
Serum	The clear fluid left after a blood clot has formed and the red and white cells have been removed – often confused with plasma (see above). Chemical analyses on blood almost always use serum or plasma and only very rarely whole blood
Specific/specificity	How good a method/technique is at disitnguishing between the substance of interest and all other substances. Absolute specificity is exceedingly difficult to achieve and most claims to have done so are usually disproved after further investigation
Stuporose	A condition in which a patient, though conscious and just able to respond to stimuli, does not do so spontaneously

Name (abbreviation)	Comment
Type 1 and type 2 diabetes	The modern way of classifying the two different types of diabetes. In patients with type 1 diabetes the insulin-secreting cells of the pancreas are destroyed and these patients are dependent on pharmaceutical insulin to stay alive. Patients with type 2 diabetes have abnormal insulin-secreting cells and ordinarily cannot produce enough insulin to keep their blood glucose levels under control without assistance
Sulphonylureas (sulphas)	A class of medicines that are taken by mouth and used to treat patients with type 2 diabetes. They stimulate the patient's own pancreas to secrete insulin even if the blood glucose concentration is already low
Unit (U)	Before insulin could be measured by weight it was measured in arbitrary units that were agreed upon internationally. Now that insulin has been obtained as a pure substance, we know that 1 milligram of it is the equivalent of 28 units; alternatively 1 unit of insulin weighs 35.7 µg.
Vomit	The expulsion of all or part of the contents of the stomach or upper intestine through the mouth

Further reading

General

Archbold GP, Southgate HJ, Teale JD, Marks V. False elevation of serum thyroxine in myxoedema due to thyroxine-binding autoantibodies. A diagnostic pitfall. *Ulster Med J* 1986; **55**: 74–9.

Bauman WA, Yalow RS. Insulin as a lethal weapon. *J Forensic Sci* 1981; **26**: 594–8.

Cryer PE. *Hypoglycemia; Pathophysiology, Diagnosis and Treatment.* Oxford: Oxford University Press, 1997: 184.

Ferner R, Norman E. *Forensic Pharmacology; Medicines, Mayhem and Malpractice.* Oxford: Oxford University Press, 1996.

Fletcher SM. Insulin. A forensic primer. *J Forensic Sci Soc* 1983: **23**: 5–17.

Galen RS, Gambino SR. *Beyond normality; The Predictive Value and Efficiency of Medical Diagnoses.* New York: Wiley, 1975.

Gatt JA, Matthewman P. Autobrewing; fact or fantasy? *Sci Justice* 2000; **40**: 211–15.

Hood I, Mirchandani H, Monforte J, Stacer W. Immunohistochemical demonstration of homicidal insulin injection site. *Arch Pathol Lab Med* 1986: **110**: 973–4.

Koskinen PJ, Nuutinen HM, Laaksonen H, et al. Importance of storing emergency serum samples for uncovered murder with insulin. *Forensic Sci Int* 1999; **105**: 61–6.

Kwong PYP, Teale JD. Screening for sulphonylureas in the investigation of hypoglycaemia. *J R Soc Med* 2002: **95**: 381–5.

Lutz R, Pedal T, Wetzel C, Mattern R. Insulin injection sites: morphology and immunochemistry. *Forensic Sci Int* 1997; **90**: 93–101.

Marks V. Forensic aspects of hypoglycaemia. In: Frier B, Fisher M (eds). *Hypoglycaemia and Diabetes.* London: Edward Arnold, 1993.

Marks V. Murder by insulin. *Med Leg J* 1999; **67**: 147–63.

Marks V. Hypoglycaemia: accidents, violence and murder, Parts 1 and 2: *Practical Diabet Int* 2005; **22**: 303–6, 352–8.

Marks V, Medd WE. Alcohol-induced hypoglycaemia. *Br J Psychiatry* 1964; **110**: 228–32.

Marks V, Rose FC. *Hypoglycaemia,* 2nd edn. Oxford: Blackwell Science, 1981: 521.

Marks V, Teale JD. Hypoglycemic disorders. *Clin Lab Med* 2001; **21**: 79–97.

Marks V, Teale JD. Drug induced hypoglycaemia. *Endocrinol Metab Clin North Am* 1999: **28**: 555–77.

Peschel O, Betz P, Eisenmenger W. Injection of toxic agents; an unusual cause of death. *Forensic Sci Int* 1995; **75**: 95–100.

Redmond JB, Nuttall FQ. Autoimmune hypoglycaemia. *Endocrinol Metab Clin North Am* 1999; **28**: 603–717.

Samols E, Marks V. Insulin assays in insulinoma. *BMJ* 1963; **i**: 507–10.

Stocklin R, Vu L, Vadas L, et al. A stable isotope dilution assay for in vivo determination of insulin levels in humans by mass-spectrometry. *Diabetes* 1997; **46**: 44–50 .

Teale JD, Wark G, Marks V. The biochemical investigation of cases of hypoglycaemia: an assessment of the clinical effectiveness of analytical services. *J Clin Pathol* 2002; **55**: 503–7 .

Kenneth Barlow

Birkinshaw VJ, Gurr MR, Randall SS, Curry AS, Price DE, Wright PH. Investigations in a case of murder by insulin poisoning: *BMJ* 1958: **ii**: 463–8.

Bathurst ME, Price DE. *Regina v Kenneth Barlow. Med Leg J* 1958; **26**: 58–71.

Herr Breslau

Janitzki U et al. Uber den Insulinnachweis in der Leiche bei Insulinvergiftung. *Med Experimentalis* 1960; **3**: 17–24.

Janitzki U et al. Uber den Insulinnachweis in der Leiche bei Insulinvergiftung 2 Mitteilung. *Med Experimentalis* 1960; **3**: 24–32.

Pfeiffer EF et al. Hypoglycemia in diabetics. In: Andreani D, Lefebvre P, Marks V (eds). *Hypoglycemia:* Stuttgart: Thieme, 1976: 112–25.

William Archerd

Bovsun M. Justice story. *New York Daily News* 15th December 2002. http://www.nydailynews.com.

People v *Archerd* (1970) 3 C3d 615 (Crim. 13053; Cal Sup Ct; Dec 10. 1970). http://online.ceb.com/calcases/C3/3C3d615.htm (accessed 18/07/06).

Pitchess P J. Proof of murder by insulin – a medico-legal first. *FBI Law Enforcement Bull* 1969; **Jan**: 16–19.

Claus von Bulow

Dershowitz A. *Reversal of Fortune*: New York: Random, 1986.

Puccio T. *In the Name of the Law: Confessions of a Trial Lawyer*. New York.WW Norton, 1995.

Dolores Christina Miller

Haibach H, Dix J D, Shah J H. Homicide by insulin administration. *J Forensic Sci* 1987; **32**: 208–16.

Levy WJ, Gardner D, Moseley J, Dix J, Gaede SE. Unusual problems for the physician in managing a hospital patient who received a malicious insulin overdose. *Neurosurgery* 1985; **17**: 992–6.

Beverly Allitt

Askill J, Sharpe M. *The Angel of Death*. London: Michael O'Mara Books, 1993.

Clothier C. *The Allitt Inquiry*. London: HMSO, 1994.

Damages victory for victim of child killer. *The Guardian* 20th July 1999.

Maria Whiston

198 *Whiston* v *Whiston* Court of Appeal [1995] 3 W.KL.R. 405.

Langford M. Main story. *Birmingham Post* Friday 23rd May 1997.

Regina v *Maria Modesta Victoria Whiston* Court of Criminal Appeal: Criminal Division No. 199704152/Z3 (Westlaw 2000 WL 1027034 (CA (Crim Div)).

Susan Shickle

R v *Shickle* Court of Appeal (Criminal Division) 14th July 2005; [2005] EWCA Crim 1881; 2005 WL 1942177.

R v *Susan Shickle* Court of Appeal (Criminal Division) Case No. 2004/02464/C3 Citation N0. [2005] EWCA Crim 1881.

Noburo Kato

Iwase H, Kobayashi M, Nakajima M, Takatori T. The ratio of insulin to C-peptide can be used to make a forensic diagnosis of exogenous insulin overdosage. *Forensic Sci Int* 2001; **115**: 123–7.

Deborah Winzar

Ben Ayed S et al. Analytical interference in hCG immunoassays: an in vivo and in vitro study. *Clin Chem 2000:* 46 (Suppl): A36.

Court of Appeal (Criminal Division) 2002: *R* v *Winzar*. All ER (D) 360 (Dec).

High Court of Justice Queens Bench Division. *R* v *Deborah Winzar* [2006] EHWC 512 (QB).

Woffinden B. A clash of convictions. *Guardian Weekend* 14th May 2005.

Vicki Jensen

The Court of Appeals of the State of Idaho: Docket No. 27465: 2002 Opinion No.16 Filed March 7th 2002: *State of Idaho* v *Vicki A. Jensen.*

Colin Bouwer

Manning PJ, Espiner EA, Yoon K, Drury PL, Holdaway IM, Bowers A. An unusual cause of hyperinsulinaemic hypoglycaemia syndrome. *Diabet Med* 2003; **20**: 772–6.

R v *Colin David Bouwer* in the High Court of New Zealand Dunedin Registry; 2001; T 70/01.

R v *Colin David Bouwer* in the Court of Appeal of New Zealand; 2002 (24th June) CA418/01. CA431/01.

Elaine Robinson

Court of Appeal Criminal Division. *R* v *Christopher Kenneth Andrews* (No. 2001 06527/X2; 2002 WL 31784552; 2002 WL 31784552 (CA (Crim Div) [2002] EWCA Crim 3021.

Index

Note: page numbers in italics are from the *Appendix*

A

Acland, Dr Peter 83
adrenocortical insufficiency 139
air injection, accident vs intent
    118–19
albumin
    insulin-induced hypoglycaemia
        125
    leakage through capillaries 114
Allitt, Beverly 55–75
    13 victims and attempted
        murders 58, 65
    arrested and released 58
    blood plasma samples analyses
        57
    Clothier Report 68
    confession 66
    first suspicions at Grantham
        Hospital 57–8
    last arrest and custody 65
    more babies admitted to QMC
        and suspension from duty
        63–5
    potassium chloride addition to
        feed 72
André, Sergeant Harry 11–12
Andrews, Chris 157–63
antibodies

auto-antibodies
    double dilution test 125,
        127–8
    interference in insulin
        measurement 124
    use in insulin measurement 13–
        14, 69–70
antidiuretic hormone, functions
    121
Archerd (Arden), Mary Brinker,
        death allegedly by road
        traffic accident 13–16
Archerd, Burney Kirk
    death by hit-and-run traffic
        accident 12–13
    suspicion of death by insulin 12
Archerd, Dorothea, possible
        victim 15
Archerd, Gladys, possible victim
        13
Archerd, Juanita
    coma attributed to barbiturate
        overdose 11
    possible victim 11–13
Archerd, William Dale (aka
        Arden, James Lynn) 9–17
    chronology of victims 10
    doubts about insulin
        measurements 16

early criminal history 9
guilty verdict and sentence 15–17
motivations for murder 16
Archerd, Zella 9–11
  death attributed to bronchopneumonia 11
Arden, James Lynn *see* Archerd, William Dale
Arquilla, Edward, Professor of Pathology 13–15
arterial (calcium) stimulation test 140–1, 150
asthma, drugs known to stimulate insulin secretion 73
autoimmune insulin syndrome (AIS) 124–5

B

Bagshawe, Prof. Kenneth 125
Ball, Jeffrey 100
Barlow, Elizabeth (first documented case) 1–6
Barlow, Kenneth 1–6
Bayesian logic 128
Beattie, Rodney 90
Berson, Sol 13–14
  radioimmunoassay for insulin measurement 13–14
  use of antibodies 13–14
beta-hydroxybutyrate 162
Blennerhassett, Prof. John 146–7
blood sample, haemolysis 144, 170
Bouwer, Annette (victim) 135–55
Bouwer, Colin 135–55
Bowers, Dr Andrew 139, 142, 144–5, 149
Bradley, Dr Robert, Harvard University 46

Breslau, Frau 7–8
Breslau, Wilhelm 7–8
  and mistress 8

C

C-peptide: insulin ratio 101–2
C-peptide, discovery 169
C-peptide assays 45, 67, 68, *170–1*
  check on natural vs administered insulin 69, 78, 99
  in control corpses 87
Cahill, Dr George 20, 39, 46
calcium infusion test 140, 141
cancer treatment, based on wrong immunoassay (Rufer, Jennifer) 126–7
carcinoid tumour 143
  see also insulinoma
Cary, Dr Nathaniel 115
choriocarcinoma, hCG and immunoassay tests 126–7, 131
citalopram 147
Clarke, Dr Penny 125
Clifton, Superintendent Stuart 55–8, 65–6
clonazepam 147
Clothier Report, Beverly Allitt 68
Cole, Dr Laurence 126–7
Cortivo, Dr Leo Dal, former President of the American Society of Forensic Toxicologists 39, 41
Crampton, Paul, aged 5 months 59–63, 67–70
  deteriorating condition and diagnosed with hypoglycaemia 59–60

further treatment and further
deterioration 61–2
improvement after treatment
with glucose drip 60
third hypoglycaemic attack and
blood specimen 67–70
transfer to Queen's Medical
Centre, Nottingham
62–3
recovery and discharge 63
creatinine 89
Criminal Cases Review Body,
flaws in expert evidence
132
Curry, Dr Alan, North-Eastern
Forensic Science
Laboratory 3–5

D

DeFronzo, Dr Ralph, Associate
Professor of Medicine 39,
46
Dershowitz, Alan
appeal against von Bulow
conviction 37
Reversal of Fortune 37
diabetes mellitus type-2 95–6
diazoxide 140–2
double dilution test, auto-
antibodies 125, 127–8
Dubowski, Dr Kurt, toxicologist
39–44
Dunne, Dominic, journalist 48–9

E

Eldin-Taylor, Philip 103
Ellis, Dr Peter 152
ergometrine 4

expert evidence, flaws, Criminal
Cases Review Body 132

F

fasting test 143
detection of an insulin-secreting
tumour 28–9
Fellner, Dr Marc
(endocrinologist) 27
Ferner, Dr Robin 86–8, 89
Bayesian logic 128
flunitrazepam 122
Forrest, Prof. Robert 104, 115,
128
Foster, Dr Daniel, Professor of
Internal Medicine 26, 39
Frazer, Dr Ruth 158–9

G

Gailitis, Dr Janis (family doctor)
21–7, 42
gastroduodenal artery, route for
calcium gluconate
injection 141
Geary, Dr 149
Geddes, Dr Jennian 119–20
Gemma, Mr Henry, prosecuting
lawyer 40–1
glibenclamide 147, 148, 151, 154
glipizide 147, 148
glossary 171–6
glucagon 168
reversal of coma 137
glucose physiology *165–7, 170*
glycogen deposition, evidence of
malicious insulin 74–5
Grantham, news of possible
multiple murders 55

Gurd, Dr MR, Boots drug
company 3–5

H

haemolysis (of blood sample)
144, 170
Halliday, Professor 142
Hamolsky, Dr Milton
(endocrinologist) 26
Harris, Dr Michael 114
Harvey, Norman (victim) 95–100
diabetes treatment 95–6
hCG and immunoassay tests 126–
7, 131
Heenan, Dr 147
hepatic vein, route for calcium
infusion test 141
Hiscutt, Mr Allan 97, 109, 113
Holdaway, Dr Ian
(endocrinologist) 150
Holman, Prof. Rury 90
Hull, Sir David 58
hyperinsulinaemic
hypoglycaemia, non-islet-
cell (NICHH) 139
hypoglycaemia
brain damage *170*
death from *169–70*
preventable 154
diagnosis post death 90
diet- and alcohol-related 45
factitious 83–6, 150
insulin-induced
and albumin 125
no inducement of vomiting
120
non-islet-cell
hyperinsulinaemic
(NICHH) 139
physiology *165–7*

septicaemia-induced 120, 125
symptoms *169–70*

I

immunoassay tests
validity and accuracy 126–7
wrong
compensation/damages sums
126
evidence eventually accepted
131
injection syringes
capacity and time taken for
injection of fatal dose
121–2
and needle tract marks 122
Instagel 139
insulin
autoimmune insulin syndrome
(AIS) 124–5
"between the toes" 91, 152
"brain insulin" 131
difficulty of causing death by
injection 8
measurement *170–1*
disappearance from
circulation 102
dose required to produce
death 121
hepatic vein 141
radioimmunoassay 15, 98–9
physiology *167–9*
used for body-building 129
insulin-induced hypoglycaemia,
no inducement of vomiting
120
insulin-secreting tumour
(insulinoma) 27, 84, 114
Annette Bouwer 136, 138–9,
141

arterial (calcium) stimulation test 140–1, 150
Isles, Alexandra, Claus von Bulow's mistress 32
islets of Langerhans
beta-cell hyperplasia 146, 150–1
physiology 167–8
Ismail, Dr Adel 124, 127–8

J

Japan, Noboru Kato 101–2
Jensen, Vicki 133–4
Jerreat, Dr Peter 96
Jobson, Jonathan 65
John, Dr Rhys 69, 73, 160
Johnson Dr 68
Johnson, Kevin 157–63
Jones, Jacky 157
Jones, Prof. Edward Lynn 82
Jones, William, death by insulin injection 15

K

Kato, Noburo (victim) 101–2

L

Laches, Dr Kenneth, Director of Emergency Room 33
Leadbetter, Dr Stephen 159
Lebovitz, Dr Harold, Professor of Endocrinology and Diabetes 39
lidocaine 73
liver, physiology 165–6
Lloyd, Eric (victim) 81–93

evidence of insulin administration 85
factitious hypoglycaemia 83–6
likelihood of insulin-secreting tumour 84
toxicology results 86–9
Lloyd, Karen 81–2, 92
Lowe, Mrs Dorothy 65

M

McCarthy, Dominic (Nic) (victim?) 103–32
McGinty, Frank 77–80
McKinnon, Dr Andrew 160
Manning, Dr Patrick (endocrinologist) 142–3, 144, 150
Marks, Prof. Vincent *(author)* 39, 42–5
Mason, Dr George 95
mass spectroscopy 131–2
Matsiko, Dr Katona 105, 112, 116
Meier, Dr Gerhard 33, 35
Meredith, Dr Emma 158, 158
metformin ("unbelievably high concentration") 147, 148, 151
Miller, Dolores Christina 51–4
actions before Erroll's death 53
actions on day of Erroll's death 52
cause of Erroll's death 54
guilty verdict 54
judge's ruling 53–4
murder accusation 52
no blood tests for insulin and C-peptide 53
suspected of killing Erroll by injecting insulin 52
Miller, Erroll 51–4

admission to hospital for
surgery on brain tumour
51
death 51–2
low blood glucose level and
treatment 51
social and medical history 51
More, David (barrister) 136, 155
Morgan, Prof. Dr Linda 89, 92
Morrison, Dr, arterial (calcium)
stimulation test 140–1

N

Nanayakkara, Dr Charithanandra
58, 71
Nash, Mark 95
nesidioblastosis 67–8
non-islet-cell hyperinsulinaemic
hypoglycaemia (NICHH)
139

O

octreotide 84, 142
inhibition of insulin secretion
84, 142
Okagbue, Mr Ernest 109–10
O'Keefe, Steven 157
Owen, Dr Philip 86
Owens, Prof. David 92

P

pancreatic beta-cell hyperplasia
146
pancreatin (enzyme) 144
Pauls, Autumn 133–4
Pearson, Matthew 133–4

Peck, Claire, aged 15 months 63–
70
emergency room treatment 64
re-admission to Grantham
Hospital w. status
asthmaticus 63–4
respiration stopped and death
64
blood analysis high
potassium levels 65
petrol and insulin injections 8
Pfeiffer, Prof. Ernst 7–8
Philips, Becky (victim) 58, 70–4
800 x expected level of insulin
71
Philips, Katie (victim) 70–4
compensation award for brain
damage 78
Pines, Dr Kermit
(endocrinologist) 28
Porter, Dr Frederick 58, 64–5, 68
potassium
level, evidence of no insulin
injection 121
plasma assay 65
Price, Dr David, Home Office
consultant pathologist 1–4
pro-insulin, check on natural vs
administered insulin 69,
169
Puccio, Thomas, trial lawyer 37,
39, 42, 44

R

radioimmunoassay, for insulin
measurement 15, 98–9
Ratnayakara, Dr 64–5
Ray, Aleta (victim) 133–4
Reeves, Dr Mark 140
Reversal of Fortune, (film) 37

Roberts, Dr 107–11
Robinson, Elaine (manslaughter victim) 157–63
Rubenstein, Prof. Dr Arthur 39, 87
Rufer, Jennifer 126–7

S

Sargeant, Nurse 64
Sarvesvaran, Dr Joseph 95–7
Schrallhammer, Maria, Sunny von Bulow's maid 46
Shickle, Andrew 97–8
Shickle, Susan 95–100
  accusation of Andrew's part in murder 100
  sentence and appeal 95–100
Steiner, Donald (C-peptide) 169
Stephens, PC Stephanie 82
Stevens, Anne (barrister) 136, 155
Stewart, Frank (Juanita Archerd's ex-husband, victim of Archerd) 11–13
  accidental death verdict 11–13
Stock, Dr Richard, family doctor 27–8, 41–3, 45
suicide?, Jane Wagstaffe 77–80
sulphasalazine 151
sulphonylureas 138, 147–50, 153–4

T

Taylor, Liam 74–5
Teale, Dr Derrick
  Beverly Allitt trial 55–7, 68–9, 71–2
  Eric Lloyd 84, 88
  Jane Wagstaffe 79

Nic McCarthy 103–4, 112–13, 128
  Norman Harvey 98
Thomas, Dr Grace, testimony at Archerd trial 16
thymoma 146
Tien, Dr 24
Tokyo, Noburo Kato 101–2
Toseland, Dr Patrick 100
Tranquada, Prof. Dr Robert 16
Turner, Prof. Robert 90

V

ventriculo–peritoneal shunt 145, 146
vitreous humour, inappropriate blood sample 78
vomiting, not in insulin-induced hypoglycaemia 120
von Bulow, Alexander, Sunny von Bulow's son 44
von Bulow, Claus 19–49
  acquittal and civil litigation by stepchildren 48
  expert evidence at trials 37–49
  history 19
  immunoassay and insulin inducing hypoglycaemia 48
  present life 49
  travesty of first trial and guilty verdict 20
von Bulow, Sunny 19–49
  first admission to hospital for hypoglycaemia 20–7
  blood and urine tests 22
  clinical notes and requirements in court of law 23

contradictory evidence of
unconsciousness 24
Decadron and Mefoxin 22,
24–5
diagnosis of hypoglycaemia
related to alcohol and
possibly barbiturates 25
diagnosis of toxic reaction 23
glucose treatment and
measurement 23–5
initial treatments for
unconciousness 22
laboratory tests, inadequacy
of 25–7
possible causes, insulin-
secreting tumour and
sulphonylurea ingestion 27
recovery and discharge 24–5,
27
time course of events 25
interim investigations 27–30
admission to investigate
cause of hypoglycaemia
27–30
alcohol, secobarbital and
tranquillizer use 29
alcohol drinking denial 30
ataxia, slurred speech and
drowsiness noticed by
family 28
discharge from hospital with
diagnosis of reactive
hypoglycaemia 30
fasting test for detection of
an insulin-secreting
tumour 28–9
glucose tolerance test 28
intravenous tolbutamide test
29
ultrasound scan, CT scan and
an arteriogram of the
pancreas 29

laboratory findings and false
suspicion of crime 35–7
blood tests 35–6
insulin and C-peptide tests 36
results falsely
suggesting murder by
insulin injection 36–7
lifestyle causing brain
damage 36–7
test for detection of
antibodies against insulin
36
life history 19, 49
medical history 19, 20–37
second emergency admission
30–2
aspirin overdose diagnosed
31–2
events during coma 35
glucose test for
hypoglycaemia 30–1
head injury annd examination
by neurosurgeon 31
no psychiatric support in
spite of suicide attempt 32
third and final emergency
admission to hospital 32–4
alcohol, amobarbital and
propranolol taken 33
blood and urine tests 33–4
breathing stopped and
resuscitated 33
diagnosis of brain damage
caused by hypoglycaemia
34
heart apparently stopped with
hypothermia 32–3
hypoglycaemic coma 19–20
transferred to Harvard
Medical School still
unconscious 34
treatment for shock 33

W

Wagstaffe, Jane, case of suicide?
    77–80
Walshe, Dr Anne (lover of Colin
    Bouwer) 148, 152
Whiston, Maria 81–93
    bigamy 91
    conviction and appeal 92–3
    order of payment of ancillary
        relief 91
Whiston, Robert 91
White, Sergeant (later Lt White)
    12–13
Wills, Mr Alan 65
Winzar, Deborah (Dee) (wrongful
    conviction?) 103–32
    trial and appeal 117–32
Wood, Dr Peter 125

Woodhead, Dr Stuart 92
Worthington, Dr Jeremy,
    neurosurgeon 34
Wright, Dr Peter
    Guy's Hospital 4
    radioactive glucose, uptake
        measurement 4

Y

Yalow, Rosalyn
    and "brain insulin" 131
    Nobel Prize for invention of
        radioimmunoassay for
        insulin measurement 13,
        69
Yoon, Dr Han-Seung 142–3, 145–
    7, 150